ALLE · ZEIT · WACH
1842

Right Hemisphere Contributions to Lexical Semantics

Edited by
Christine Chiarello

With 25 Figures

Springer-Verlag Berlin Heidelberg New York
London Paris Tokyo

Christine Chiarello, Ph. D.
Syracuse University
College of Arts and Sciences
Department of Psychology
430 Huntington Hall, 150 Marshall Street
Syracuse, NY, 13244-2340/USA

ISBN-13:978-3-642-73676-6 e-ISBN-13:978-3-642-73674-2
DOI: 10.1007/978-3-642-73674-2

Library of Congress Cataloging-in-Publication Data. Right hemisphere contributions to lexical semantics/edited by Christine Chiarello.p.cm.Includes index.ISBN-13:978-3-642-73676-6(U.S.) 1. Semantics–Psychological aspects. 2. Neuropsychology. 3. Psycholinguistics. 4. Cerebral hemispheres. 5. Brain-Localization of functions. I. Chiarello, Christine. P325.5.P78R5 1988 612'.825–dc19 88-19975

Softcover reprint of the hardcover 1st edition 1988

2125/3130-543210 Printed on acid-free paper

Preface

Language depends on a normally functioning left hemisphere. This central fact of human cerebral dominance was well established by 19th century aphasiologists and has been repeatedly confirmed by subsequent investigations. Predominance, however, does not imply exclusivity. As demonstrated by the commissurotomy patients studied by Eran Zaidel and associates, the right hemisphere is also capable of subserving some linguistic functions. The question, then, is not *whether* the right hemisphere can process language, but how and when it does so.

This volume focuses on the right hemisphere's contribution to one important aspect of language, lexical semantics. Although the right hemisphere may well be involved in other linguistic functions, such as prosody, the greatest evidence for right hemisphere language competence has been obtained for the processing of word meanings. In addition, cognitive psychology and psycholinguistics have provided us with well-developed models of the lexicon and lexical access to guide our inquiry. Finally, there are techniques available for studying lateralized lexical processing in the normal as well as in the brain-injured hemispheres. For these reasons, a focus on the lexicon is likely to yield the greatest number of insights about right-hemisphere language processing.

This volume represents a sampling of some of the most intriguing research done recently on right-hemisphere lexical processing. Although no attempt is made to exhaustively survey this field, data from right-brain injured (Joanette and Goulet; Brownell), left-brain injured (Landis and Regard; Weniger, Kitteringham, and Eglin), and normal individuals (Chiarello; Zaidel, White, Sakurai, and Banks) is included. It is interesting that Zaidel and colleagues have chosen to present their work on normal subjects, rather than the commissurotomy patients. While the split-brain data has been important in directing attention to the possibility of a right-hemisphere lexicon, it should be clear that the evidence for right-hemisphere language processing does not hinge on any particular interpretation of the "representativeness" of data obtained from a few, carefully selected commissurotomy cases.

The individual chapters provide evidence that the right hemisphere may be involved in a wide variety of lexical semantic functions and document the conditions under which right hemisphere participation may occur. Joanette and Goulet discuss a possible role for the right hemisphere in language production by carefully delineating the impairments shown by right hemisphere-injured patients in semantic fluency tests. Brownell demonstrates a deficit in the appreciation of metaphoric alternative word meanings following right hemisphere damage and relates this to previous work, showing impairments among such patients in understanding nonliteral, connotative aspects of meaning. Landis and Regard present case studies of right-hemisphere reading after left-hemisphere injury and interpret this data in terms of a model of interhemispheric inhibition and release. Weniger et al. investigate word reading in global aphasic patients and find the greatest evidence for right hemisphere participation among the most severely aphasic individuals.

Both Chiarello and Zaidel et al. investigate right hemisphere lexical semantics in normal subjects using visual half-field techniques. Chiarello reports the results of semantic priming experiments which suggest that the right hemisphere may maintain a set of alternate meanings via automatic semantic facilitation, while the left hemisphere focuses on a single interpretation. Zaidel et al. investigate the hemispheric basis of several lexical congruity effects (Stroop, semantic priming, comparative judgments). They argue that such effects cannot be properly interpreted without considering the separate contributions of the left and right hemispheres. In a final chapter Milberg critically evaluates the findings of each investigator with respect to the assumptions made about representation and control functions of each hemisphere. In so doing he outlines the requirements for a theory of right-hemisphere lexical semantic processing.

The studies reported here relate to a current controversy about the use of neuropsychological data in theory construction. It is becoming increasingly common for cognitive neuropsychologists to assert that delineation of the neural structures which subserve various cognitive functions is irrelevant if the goal is to construct and test well-defined processing models. Neuropsychological data, then, is important in order to demonstrate processing dissociations, but the nature/location of the brain dysfunction producing such dissociations is not germane. The authors contributing to this volume, by virtue of their interest in the *right-hemisphere* semantic system, have implicitly rejected this view. As the research reported here attests, there are both quantitative and qualitative differences in how the left and right hemispheres process word meaning. Ultimately, cognitive models must incorporate these differences or run the risk of failing to capture a salient property of the human mind.

Earlier versions of the chapters by Brownell, Chiarello, Joanette and Goulet, and Zaidel et al. were presented at a symposium entitled "Defining the Right Hemisphere's Contribution to Lexical Semantics" held in Veldhoven, The Netherlands, on June 27, 1986, as part of the ninth annual European meeting of the International Neuropsychological Society. William Milberg served as the discussant. The interest generated by this symposium encouraged us to solicit additional contributions for a published volume. Special thanks to Dorothea Weniger for bringing this work to the attention of the publishers, and to Dr. Thomas Thiekötter, Ms. Stephanie Benko, and Mr. G. Schulze of Springer-Verlag for their kind assistance.

Syracuse, July 1988 CHRISTINE CHIARELLO

Contents

List of Contributors

WILLIAM BANKS, Department of Psychology, Pomona College, Claremont, California 91711 USA

HIRAM H. BROWNELL, Department of Psychology, Boston College, Chestnut Hill, Massachusetts, 02167 USA

CHRISTINE CHIARELLO, Department of Psychology, Syracuse University, Syracuse, New York 13244-2340 USA

MIRJAM EGLIN, Institute of Cognitive Studies, University of California, Berkeley, California 94720 USA

PIERRE GOULET, Laboratoire Théophile-Alajouanine, Centre de Recherche, CHCN, 4565, Chemin de la Reine-Marie, Montréal, Quebec, Canada H3W 1W5

YVES JOANETTE, Laboratoire Théophile-Alajouanine, Centre de Recherche, CHCN, 4565, Chemin de la Reine-Marie, Montréal, Quebec, Canada H3W 1W5

VIVIAN KITTERINGHAM, Department of Neurology, University of Zürich, Frauenklinikstrasse 26, 8091 Zürich, Switzerland

THEODOR LANDIS, Department of Neurology, University of Zürich, Frauenklinikstrasse 26, 8091 Zürich, Switzerland

WILLIAM MILBERG, Geriatric Research, Education and Clinical Center, V.A. Medical Center, 1400 VFW Parkway, West Roxbury, Massachusetts 02132 USA

MARIANNE REGARD, Department of Neurology, University of Zürich, Frauenklinikstrasse 26, 8091 Zürich, Switzerland

ERIKO SAKURAI, Department of Psychology, University of California, Los Angeles, California 90024-1563 USA

DOROTHEA WENIGER, Department of Neurology, University of Zürich, Frauenklinikstrasse 26, 8091 Zürich, Switzerland

Hedy White, Department of Psychology, Western Carolina University, Cullowhee, North Carolina 28723 USA

Eran Zaidel, Department of Psychology, University of California, Los Angeles, California 90024-1563 USA

Word-Naming in Right-Brain-Damaged Subjects *

Yves Joanette and Pierre Goulet

Introduction

The mere fact this book addresses the question of the right hemisphere's contribution to lexical semantics bears in itself a strong, and widely accepted, hypothesis; that is, if the right hemisphere contributes to any of the cognitive processes necessary for language, lexicosemantic ones are probably among the most likely. This assumption proceeds from an amazingly large number of studies using different experimental paradigms. Of these, the analysis of the linguistic capacities of the right hemisphere in split-brain patients can probably be considered as having been one of the most productive. Indeed, not only did these studies provide some evidence for the linguistic capacities of the right hemisphere as far as lexical semantics are concerned, but they also stimulated research with normal subjects using, for example, hemifield studies. From studies with split-brain and normal subjects it can be inferred that the right hemisphere of right-handers has some lexicosemantic capacity which is, at least quantitatively and probably even qualitatively, different from that of the left hemisphere. One can summarize this capacity by saying that it is optimal for the comprehension of frequent and concrete lexical items (Beaumont 1982; Bradshaw et al. 1977; Bradshaw and Nettleton 1983; Chiarello 1985; Gazzaniga 1983; Gazzaniga and Hillyard 1978; Gazzaniga and Sperry 1967; Hannequin et al. 1987; Millar and Whitaker 1983; Searleman 1983; Zaidel 1983). However, all these studies point essentially to the fact that the right hemisphere of right-handers has some specific lexicosemantic *potential*. Given this potential, the question is whether or not the right hemisphere really *contributes* to lexicosemantic function when it is normally connected to the left hemisphere.

Studies of the performance of right-brain-damaged right-handers (RBD) given a lexicosemantic task represent one way of looking at the real contribution of the right hemisphere to lexical semantics. Apart from the general question stated above, and given a positive answer to this question, a more specific way of stating the problem is to ask, for which lexicosemantic processes or set of processes is the integrity of the right hemisphere necessary? A certain number of studies have shown RBD subjects' performance to be affected when

* This research was supported by program grant PG-28 of the Conseil de recherches médicales du Canada as well as by grants from the Fonds de la recherche en santé du Québec and Fonds de recherche et de développement de l'Université de Montréal.

given lexicosemantic tasks (Gainotti et al. 1983; Lesser 1974). But these studies essentially give information as to the importance of the integrity of the right hemisphere for *understanding* lexical items. Under these conditions, subjects typically have to (a) *refer* to semantic knowledge and (b) express, verbally or not, some opinion or judgment. Thus, this does not tell us if the right hemisphere's integrity is actually necessary when this semantic knowledge is *used* actively in the context of a task requiring verbal production, a condition which is closer to what an individual actually has to do in the context of natural production. Such a task is the focus of the present paper.

Here again, there are probably many means by which one can evaluate the importance of the integrity of the right hemisphere for the implementation of lexicosemantic processes in the context of active production. One of these is a *word-naming* or *verbal fluency* task. Such a task has been used in the past as a mean of evaluating overall productivity in brain-lesioned patients (Milner 1964; Thurstone 1938), particularly in patients with frontal damage who show lack of spontaneity or initiative (Hécaen and Albert 1978). However, this task also allows an on-line glimpse of those lexicosemantic processes. Since word-naming criteria can be qualitatively different, the effectiveness of different lexical exploration and retrieval can be compared; for example, the nature of the lexical exploration induced by formal criteria is probably not the same as that induced by semantic criteria. Moreover, qualitative analyses of the word-naming performance can give some information on the way right-brain-damaged subjects explore and access lexicosemantic knowledge. Such a description can also give some indication of the exact structure of the lexicon available to the right hemisphere, or else of the nature of the lexical access of the right hemisphere, if it is considered that both hemispheres do indeed access the same lexicon. In doing so, it is possible to draw some inferences about the exact nature of the normal right hemisphere's contribution to those cognitive processes necessary for lexicosemantic functioning. Hence, the present chapter reports a series of studies using the word-naming task paradigm with right-brain-damaged subjects.

A certain number of studies in the literature have focused directly on word-naming performance in RBD subjects, though more frequently information has been a by-product of some other interest. However, there are also a considerable number of contradictions between results of these studies, probably because there are many methodological differences between them. For example, word-naming criteria and production time allowed can be very different from one study to another. An even more confounding factor is that these studies are not comparable with respect to the etiology or the localization of right-brain lesions. In other words, there is no clear-cut answer as to whether or not right-brain damage affects performance on a word-naming task. The goal of the first study reported here (Study I) is to investigate whether RBD subjects word-naming performance is affected, thus providing some support for the possibility of an actual right-hemisphere contribution to lexicosemantic processes. Given that word-naming performance is indeed affected, then subsequent goals of the first study are to determine if some methodological aspects concerning both the word-naming criteria and lesion-related parameters can explain the discrepancies observed between results of previous studies. Based on the results of Study I, qualitative analyses of right-brain-damaged subjects' word-naming production were conducted in two subsequent studies. One of these studies (Study II) was devised to look for factors that could account for RBD subjects' reduction in word-naming performance as well as to investigate whether this reduction was present throughout the task. The final study (Study III) focused on a description of right-brain-damaged subjects' lexical exploration strategy.

Study I: Criterion-Specific Reduction of Word-Naming Performance

Previous studies which investigated word-naming performance in right-brain-damaged subjects have employed either a formal criterion (i.e., words beginning with a given letter, such as the FAS test) or a semantic one (i.e., words referring to a given superordinate, such as animal names). Using formal criteria, a certain number of studies did report RBD-subjects to demonstrate reduced word-naming performance as compared to normal controls (Bolter et al. 1983; Borkowski et al. 1967; Bruyer and Tuyumbu 1980; Perret 1974; Ramier and Hécaen 1970), despite contradictory results by Benton (1968). However, most of these studies were conducted in such a manner that it is not possible to state whether this reduction results from the lesion being in the *right* hemisphere or, alternatively, the lesion being *frontal* (Bruyer and Tuyumbu 1980; Ramier and Hécaen 1970), or the nature of the lesion (e.g., a tumor) perhaps having been associated with left-hemisphere dysfunction (Bolter et al. 1983; Borkowski et al. 1967; Perret 1974). Furthermore, results of studies using *semantic* criteria are very contradictory; Boller (1968) found RBD subjects to perform worse than controls, whereas Grossman (1981) did not find such a difference.

Moreover, the exact significance of these two studies is complicated not only by the fact that Boller (1968) gives no indication as to the etiology of the lesion, but also that the criteria employed do not appear to be comparable in the two studies. Indeed, whereas Boller (1968) used only one broad semantic criterion (animal names), Grossman (1981) used different semantic criteria, including some much narrower (e.g., bird names).

Thus, it is difficult to know whether or not word-naming is indeed affected in right-handers with a lesion limited to the right hemisphere. Given the fact that all the evidence concerning the contribution of the right hemisphere to lexical semantics pertains to semantic processing, and considering the systematic absence of impairments at the formal level (Gazzaniga 1983; Lesser 1974), one could suggest that if word-naming is indeed affected in RBD subjects, it should be more so when criteria are semantic rather than formal. Hence, it is hypothesized that the right hemisphere essentially contributes to proper semantic processes implicated in lexical semantics. The goal of Study I is to verify this hypothesis while, at the same time, controlling for both (a) restrictiveness of the right-hemisphere dysfunction by including only patients with vascular etiology and (b) the frontal character of the lesion.

Method

Subjects. The subjects were 55 French-speaking adult right-handers, i.e., having obtained at least +80 on the Edinburgh Handedness Inventory (Oldfield 1971). Thirty-five of these subjects had suffered single unilateral vascular lesion to the right hemisphere (RBD subjects). Another 20 subjects, although ill and hospitalized, had no neurological insult (C subjects).

There was no significant difference between RBD and C subjects as to mean age [57.1 and 56.8 respectively for C and RBD subjects; $t(53)=0.09$, N.S.], sex ratio (13♂/7♀ and 24♂/11♀ respectively for C and RBD subjects; corrected chi-square=0.0, $df=1$, N.S.), presence/absence of a familial history of left-handedness or ambidexterity (6/14 and 9/26 respectively for C and RBD subjects; corrected chi-square=0.0, $df=1$, N.S.), mean number of years of education [8.3 and 8.8 years respectively for C and RBD subjects; $t(53)=0.5$, N.S.] and presence/absence of second language abilities (8/12 and 22/13 respectively for C and RBD subjects; corrected chi-square=1.84, $df=1$, N.S.).

Word-Naming Task and Procedure. Subjects were required within a two-minute period to orally produce the greatest number of words according to one of the following four criteria:

- Formal criteria: words beginning with letters "B" or "R".
- Semantic criteria: words belonging to the semantic class whose superordinate is either "Animal" or "Furniture".

Each criterion was explained to the subjects and illustrated using the same two examples. All subjects had to produce words according to all four criteria. They were instructed to produce items which were different from the provided examples, not to repeat any item, and to avoid proper nouns. If a subject ceased producing items, the examiner encouraged the subject to produce more only once. Each subject's response was tape-recorded and afterwards was broadly transcribed for analysis. Only acceptable items were thereafter analyzed, i.e., items defined as the first occurrence of a French lexical item which conformed to the given criteria and which respected the task constraints.

Results

For both formal and semantic criteria, acceptable items produced according to either one of two criteria, – "B" and "R" for formal and "Animal" and

"Furniture" for semantic – were totaled; this was done since there was no significant difference between number of words produced according to each of the two formal criteria on the one hand, and between each of the two semantic criteria on the other hand. This summation reduced the experimental design to a two-factor experiment with repeated measures on one factor; the between-subjects factor, group (G), opposed C to RBD subjects, whereas the within-subject factor, criterion (C), opposed performances on the formal and the semantic criteria.

Since these results have been reported in detail elsewhere (Joanette and Goulet 1986), only those most relevant for the discussion at hand are presented here. Table 1 contains means and standard deviations of the scores for each criterion within each group. Results of an ANOVA show a significant G × C interaction effect ($F_{1,53}=4.77$; $P<0.05$). Furthermore, main effects of factors G and C are also significant: On the one hand, C subjects had higher scores than RBD subjects and, on the other hand, more acceptable items were produced on the basis of a semantic rather than a formal criterion. Analysis of the simple effects reveals the nature of the G × C interaction (Table 2); it shows RBD subjects to differ significantly from C subjects for semantic criteria only.

Table 1. Mean and standard deviation (SD) of the scores for each type of criteria within each group

Group	Criteria	Mean	SD
C	Formal	24.5	13.1
	Semantic	43.2	7.9
RBD	Formal	20.0	11.3
	Semantic	32.5	10.5

Table 2. Results of the simple effects analysis. Note that MS within cell is the average of MS (subjects within group) and MS (C × subjects within group). The degrees of freedom of the F test using MS within cell as denominator are respectively 1 and 79 (according to Winer 1971)

Simple effect	SS	df	MS	F
Criteria for group C	3515.63	1	3515.63	71.0*
Criteria for group RBD	2803.56	1	2803.56	56.6*
Criteria × Subject within groups	2625.82	53	49.54	
Groups for formal criteria	261.01	1	261.01	2.20 (N. S.)
Groups for semantic criteria	1435.82	1	1435.82	12.08*
Within cell source of variation			118.90	

* $P<0.01$

Table 3. Mean and standard deviation for each criteria within each subgroup of RBD subjects, namely RBDf and RBDnf

Group	Criteria	Mean	SD
RBDf	Formal	21.2	12.7
$n=15$	Semantic	34.3	8.9
RBDnf	Formal	19.2	13.0
$n=10$	Semantic	32.3	16.2

RBD subjects were then divided into two groups according to positive evidence of the presence (RBDf, $n=15$) or absence (RBDnf, $n=10$) of an anterior lesion. Resulting subgroups were not significantly different according to mean age [$t(23)=1.81$, $P=0.08$], sex ratio (corrected chi-square$=0.0$, $df=1$, $P=1.0$), presence/absence of a familial history of left-handedness or ambidexterity (corrected chi-square$=0.0$, $df=1$, $P=1.0$), mean number of years of education [$t(23)=0.63$, $P=0.54$] and presence/absence of second language abilities (corrected chi-square$=10.17$, $df=1$, $P=0.68$). Table 3 contains the mean scores and the standard deviations for RBDf and RBDnf groups. An ANOVA did not show any $G \times C$ interaction effect ($F1,23=0.0$; $P=0.99$). The only effect that remains significant in this analysis is the criterion effect (semantic better than formal; $F1,23=34.2$; $P<0.01$). Thus, word-naming scores do not significantly discriminate RBDf from RBDnf subjects.

Discussion

The present study yielded results that support the hypothesis being tested. RBD-subjects with lesions limited to the right hemisphere do evidence lowered word-naming performance. However, this reduction is present only when the criterion is semantic, not when it is formal. Moreover, such a reduction in word-naming cannot be attributed to a general lack of initiative, since (a) it is criterion-specific and (b) not dependent upon the frontal or nonfrontal nature of the lesion.

Given what has been said earlier, it may be that the RBD subjects in those studies which have claimed lowered word-naming performance using formal criteria (Bolter et al. 1983; Borkowski et al. 1967; Bruyer and Tuyumbu 1980; Perret 1974; Ramier and Hécaen 1970) had more than a right-hemisphere dysfunction; indeed, the nature of the lesion's etiology was not controlled for in most of them. Our results, as far as semantic criteria are concerned, do not agree with those of Grossman (1981). This might be due to the fact that Grossman (1981) used semantic criteria corresponding to much narrower semantic fields. Since a restrictive criterion is probably much less productive, it could have resulted in a ceiling effect in normal control subjects, thus masking a possible difference between normal control and RBD subjects. A similar comment could be addressed to the difference found here between formal and semantic criteria: indeed, it could be that the fact that there is no significant difference between groups of subjects with regard to formal criteria is due in part to their lowered productivity. Future studies should control for productivity when comparing formal and semantic criteria.

The present results indicate that right-hemisphere integrity is necessary for proper lexicosemantic functioning in a production task. In the present task, this contribution appears to be specific to semantic aspects per se and not to depend upon the general lack of initiation that may be associated with some right-hemisphere lesions, particularly if these are frontal. Of course, the present results do not suggest that this contribution is exclusive to the right hemisphere, nor would we like to advance such an hypothesis. On the contrary, given that both formal *and* semantic aspects of lexicosemantic processing can be affected in left-brain-damaged (LBD) aphasics, it could be hypothesized that while the integrity of both left and right hemisphere seems necessary for semantic aspects proper, the condition of left-hemisphere integrity appears sufficient for processing formal aspects of lexical-semantics. In other words, the right hemisphere seems to play a somewhat qualitatively different role than the left hemisphere in lexical semantics; the right hemisphere contributes only to semantic access to the lexicon proper, and not to its formal access. In order to further address these questions, one should look more specifically for reasons why word-naming performance is lowered among RBD subjects when the criterion is semantic.

Study II: Error Analysis and Time Course of Word-Naming Production

The goal of Study II is to identify further reasons that could account for the lowered word-naming performance of RBD subjects when the criterion is semantic, as revealed in the previous study. One aim is to see if the impairment responsible for lowered semantic word-naming performance is indeed semantic or whether it represents an artifact which would manifest itself only for semantic criteria. The first point to be investigated is the number of errors, or unacceptable items, that RBD subjects produce. Indeed, some relation could exist between a decrease in word-naming and an increase in the number of errors, such that RBD subjects produce less acceptable items only because they produce more unacceptable items. An increase in the number of errors could reveal difficulties such as problems respecting either semantic or task constraints. In some cases, such as dementia, it has been shown that subjects produce a greater number of unacceptable items while producing less acceptable items (Ober et al. 1986). It could be that for some unknown reason word-naming based on semantic criteria can be affected more.

Notwithstanding the total number of unacceptable items, the second part of this investigation pertains to error patterns. Indeed, this pattern may reveal information about the factors responsible for the word-naming reduction. It is known, for instance, that RBD subjects tend to perseverate (Marcie et al. 1965); thus, RBD subjects could produce a greater number of unacceptable items of the perseverative type. Error patterns could also reflect RBD subjects' semantic impairment (Bradshaw and Nettleton 1983; Coltheart 1980; Millar and Whitaker 1983; Saffran et al. 1980; Zaidel 1983); for example, problems in respecting semantic class boundaries could lead to difficulties in respecting constraints imposed by the superordinate.

The third factor that will be examined is the temporal distribution of productions in RBD subjects. At least two thoughts underlie the investigation. The first is the definite elimination of any nonspecific factor such as *asponta-neity* that could account for RBD subjects' lowered word-naming performance. Indeed, a time course analysis would indicate such a factor since, if present, word-naming would be lowered throughout the task. The second one implicates different cognitive processes involved at different periods of a word-naming task. Indeed, Rosen (1980) suggests that a word-naming task involves a two-stage process organized sequentially in time. In the first moment of a word-naming task, items produced would be those linked most directly with the superordinate itself. Thus, performance in the first moment of a naming task seems to depend on the automatic activation of items through spreading activation originating from the superordinate. After this first moment, subjects probably proceed in a more controlled fashion in order to continue word-naming. At that point subjects have to organize themselves systematically. In other words, the first moment of a word-naming task appears dependent on automatic activation of the lexicon, whereas the postinitial moments seem to involve less automatic and more organized exploration of the same lexicon. Thus, the time course of word production for semantic criteria of RBD subjects will be compared to that of C subjects in order to further clarify the nature of RBD subjects' impairments within these two time constraints.

Method

Details of this study are found in Joanette et al. (1988). Subjects and procedures are the same as described in Study I except that only lexical items produced for semantic criteria were considered here. These items were identified as either "acceptable" or "unacceptable". Acceptable items were defined as the first occurrence of a French lexical item which respected the task criteria. All the other items were labelled as unacceptable and classified as follows:

- the production of a word not fully respecting the given criterion (nonrespect errors)
- the repetition of an item (repetition errors)

– the production of one of the examples given by the examiner (example errors)
– the production of nonwords, i.e., items not recognized as lexical items in French (non-word errors)

Results

Number of Errors. Results show that there is no significant difference between the number of unacceptable items produced by RBD and C subjects for semantic criteria; $t(53) = 0.44$, N.S.

Pattern of Error Types. All except a few unacceptable items have been labeled according to one of the four predefined error types. Figure 1 shows the distribution of error types for both groups of subjects for semantic criteria. The pattern of errors is quite similar for C and RBD subjects. A t test yields no significant difference as far as number of repetitions [$t(53) = 0.96$, N.S.] and non-respect [$t(53) = 0.29$, N.S.] errors are concerned. Given that the subjects made very few errors of the other types, a chi-square was used. These comparisons reveal no significant difference for number of example errors ($\chi^2 = 0.92$, N.S.) and for number of nonword errors ($\chi^2 = 1.00$, N.S.). Thus, it can be stated that there is no significant difference between the two groups in the number of each error type produced, considering each error type independently.

Time Course of Production. Figure 2 presents the number of items produced compiled for each of the four 30-s periods in the total 2-min period allowed for production for both C and RBD subjects. The total number of items produced was used for two reasons: first, it was felt that the integrity of the two postulated time-constrained sets of processes could best be evaluated by reference to subjects' total production, and secondly, it was previously shown that there is no significant difference between the two groups with regard to number of unacceptable items.

The effects of the group (G) and of the time period (TP) over the number of total items produced by subjects were examined using an ANOVA with a 2×4 (G $\times$ TP) factorial design with repeated measures on the second factor.

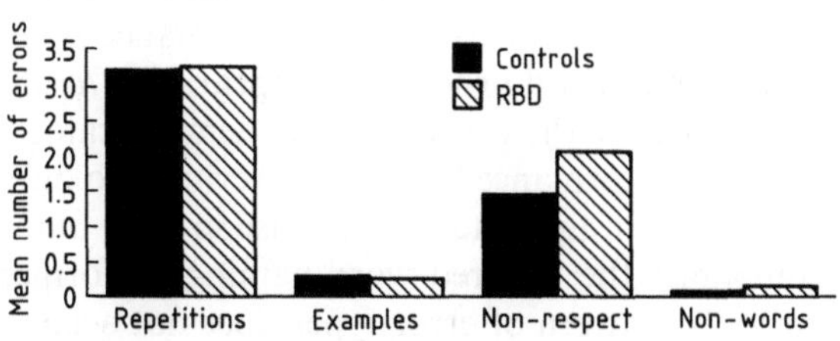

Fig. 1. Mean number of errors according to types for C and RBD subjects

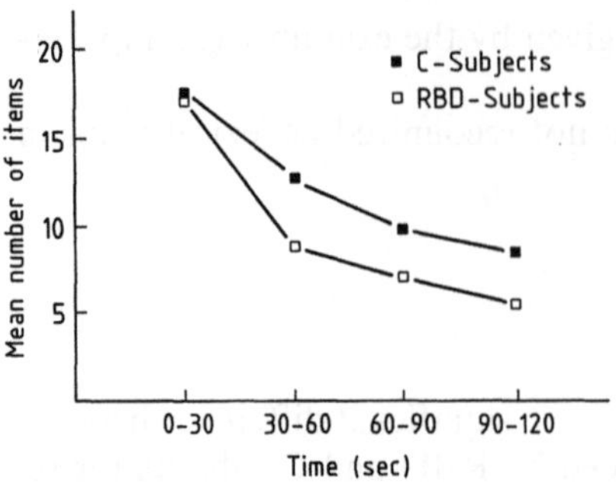

Fig. 2. Mean number of items produced by C and RBD subjects according to semantic criteria, presented for each of the four 30-s periods included in the 2-min period time allowed for production

Results show a practically significant G × TP interaction effect ($F3,159 = 2.63$; $P = 0.052$). Main effects of factors G and TP are also significant: on the one hand, C subjects produce more items than RBD subjects ($F1,53 = 11.91$; $P < 0.001$), and, on the other hand, both groups of subjects produce a greater number of words at the beginning of the allowed production time ($F3,159 = 93.18$; $P < 0.001$). Indeed, Fig. 2 shows that, on the whole, more items are produced within the first 30-s period than the second 30-s period, more items are produced during the second than within the third 30-s period, and so forth.

A simple effects analysis for the TP factor reveals the exact nature of the interaction between G and TP. Indeed, RBD subjects produce a significantly smaller number of items than C subjects for all periods ($P < 0.05$) except during the first 30-s period ($P = 0.30$).

Discussion

Results show that RBD subjects' lowered word-naming performance for semantic criteria is not accompanied by a corresponding increase in the number of unacceptable items. Moreover, the patterns of errors are, on the whole, similar for RBD and C subjects. However, a time course analysis reveals that the difference between RBD and C subjects' word-naming performance is not present in the first 30-s period. Indeed, significant difference between RBD and C subjects' word-naming performance is essentially to be attributed to a reduction in word production appearing *after* the first 30-s period.

Results of the error analysis demonstrate RBD subjects' lowered word-naming performance for semantic criteria to differ from that of demented subjects, since in the latter an increase in total number of unacceptable items accompanies the lowered word-naming performance (Ober et al. 1986). Similarly, the pattern of error types does not account for RBD subjects' lowered word-naming performance. Indeed, RBD subjects' do not produce more repetition errors, thus ruling out the possibility that a general or even a more specific perseverative behavior has interfered with the task performance, nor do they produce more nonrespect errors. This also rules out certain types of impairment in semantic organization, such as a loosening of semantic fields or an unrefrained tendency to free associate.

The results of the time course analysis are more informative. Indeed, as already mentioned, RBD subjects' lowered word-naming performance for semantic criteria is not present throughout the entire production time allowed: RBD and C subjects' performance is comparable for the first 30-s period, but thereafter RBD subjects' word-naming performance decreases rapidly and remains low for the rest of the production time. This confirms one of the conclusions of Study I: a general aspontaneity factor can be ruled out since it would have been evident throughout the whole production time.

In fact, such results could indicate that RBD subjects' word-naming performance is different according to the kind of lexical exploration required by the task. More specifically, RBD subjects seem to have few, if any, problems in the first moment of the task. It is postulated that during this phase performance is dependent on the automatic activation of a series of items directly linked with the superordinate. However, as soon as those strongly linked items are produced, subjects have to consciously organize their exploration of the lexicon in order to perform. Then the cognitive processes involved may be said to be less automatic. If such processes are effectively involved, then it could by hypothesized that RBD subjects' lowered word production for semantic criteria might be the result of lowered efficiency of those less automatic processes necessary for optimal lexicon exploration or access, and not that of a gross modification in the semantic organization itself. This explanation remains hypothetical, however, since a discrete problem in semantic organization could probably also interfere with the efficiency of those less automatic processes. Nonetheless, the integrity of the right hemisphere in normal right-handers still appears to be necessary for efficient exploration of the semantic organization and/or for the integrity of fine aspects of semantic networks on which such exploration is based.

In order to further specify this contribution, one could look at the exploration strategy used by RBD subjects. At least two complementary strategies are likely: (a) to identify [1] semantic subfields and (b) to take advantage of each subfield in an optimal fashion. The integrity of these two mechanisms is further analyzed in Study III.

---

[1] We take the term "identify" here to mean that a given subject either explicitly identifies a given superordinate, like the superordinate "farm animals", from which he then selects the different relevant semantic items, *or* that the subject "identifies" the corresponding subset by an item-by-item scanning strategy, but without the subject being explicitely aware of the particular subset he is exploring or of the particular unifying semantic link.

Study III: Semantic Clustering in Word-Naming

Whether or not these two mechanisms are indeed used by all normal individuals, optimal production in a word-naming task requires evocation of the greatest number of (a) semantic subfields, and (b) items within each semantic subfield. The goal of this study is to qualitatively analyze the production of RBD subjects in order to determine if their lowered word-naming performance is associated with either a reduced number of identified subfields, a reduced number of items produced within each subfield, or both. Moreover, some characteristics of the semantic fields activated by RBD subjects are also tentatively described by looking at the number of different items produced by each group of subjects as well as the exclusiveness of the produced items.

Method

A detailed description of the methods and results of this study are to be found elsewhere (Goulet and Joanette, in preparation). The analyses were made on the same word-naming performance used for Studies I and II, except that the responses of 5 subjects were not included since these subjects were not North American, and the present study relies upon a qualitative analysis of production in terms of semantic clusters.

Subjects' responses for the semantic criterion "animal" [2] were analyzed according to the following four parameters:

1. Number of different words produced by each group of subjects
2. Number of different words produced by one group of subjects but not by the other
3. Number of different semantic subfields referred to by each subject
4. Number of words emitted by each subject for the most exploited subfield [3]

   In the present study a *semantic subfield* is recognized when at least three consecutive animal names share a common attribute, like farm or jungle animals. According to these criteria a given word can be included in a given subfield for one subject (e.g., chicken in farm animals), but also in another subfield for another subject (e.g., chicken in animals that can fly, i.e., birds). The retained attributes were always those allowing maximal clustering, i.e., the grouping of the greatest number of at least three consecutive items. However, total number of items for a given subfield includes those items that are not necessarily consecutive to the ones which permitted the identi-

[2] This study was made only by reference to the semantic criterion "animal" since it was the only one to allow adequate clustering. Indeed, the other semantic criterion, "furniture", was such that clusters could not be identified in a unequivocal manner.

[3] All the words produced for a semantic subfield did not have to be consecutive as long as at least three of them were, thus allowing a subfield to be recognized.

fication of the subfield. Semantic subfields were determined for each subject by two independent judges.

Furthermore, the correlation between total number of words produced and the number of different subfields, on the one hand, and number of items for the most productive subfield, on the other hand, was investigated. This was done to support the postulate that production in this kind of task is related to both the identification of a maximum of different subfields and the maximal production of words for each of these subfields.

Results

Number of Different Items Produced by Each Group. As a group RBD subjects produced a smaller number of different lexical items. RBD subjects emitted 143 different animal names, among which 41 are exclusive to this group, as compared to the 174 different animal names produced by C subjects among which 72 are exclusive to this group. These results increase in significance considering the fact that the larger number of different animal names produced by the C group as well as the larger number of names exclusive to this group, come from a smaller number of subjects ($n=20$) than the RBD group ($n=30$).

Number of Semantic Subfields. For C subjects there is a significant correlation ($r=0.65$; $P<0.01$) between the number of semantic subfields emitted and the mean number of items produced for the animal criterion. However, Fig. 3 shows that RBD subjects emitted a significantly smaller number of semantic subfields than C subjects did [$T(48)=2.58$; $P<0.02$]. Indeed, whereas C subjects emitted on the average nearly six different semantic subfields, RBD subjects' production contained on the average less than four different subfields.

Number of Lexical Items Produced for the Most Exploited Subfield. For C subjects there is a significant correlation between the mean number of lexical items produced for the most productive semantic subfield and the mean number of

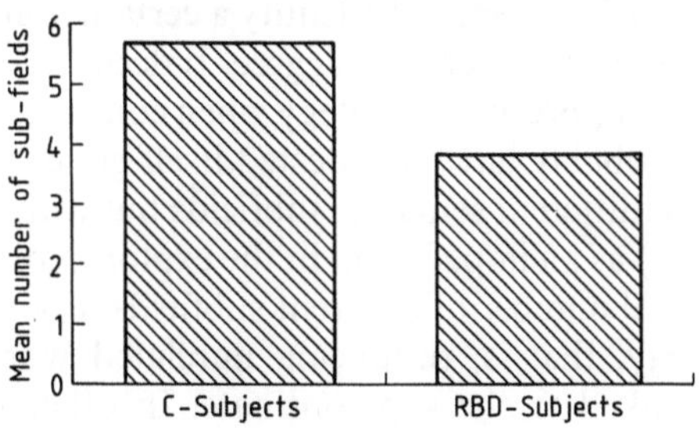

Fig. 3. Mean number of semantic subfields referred to by C and RBD subjects

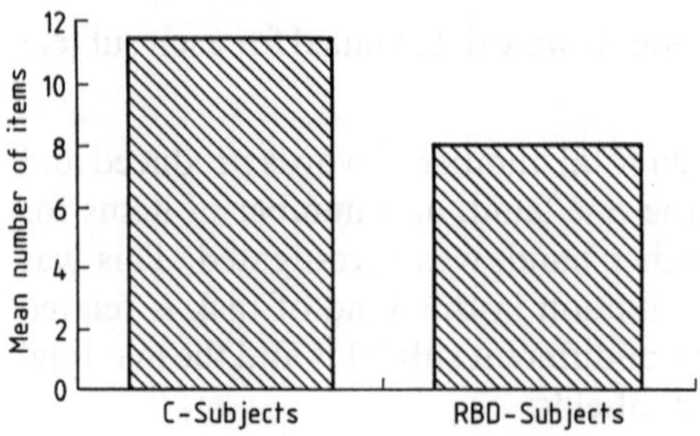

Fig. 4. Mean number of lexical items produced by C and RBD subjects for the most exploited subfield

items produced for the animal criterion. However, Fig. 4 shows that RBD subjects are, on the average, less productive than C subjects in the number of lexical items produced for the most exploited semantic subfield [T(25.62) = 2.79; $P < 0.02$]. Indeed, whereas C subjects emitted approximately 11 different animal names for their most exploited semantic subfield, RBD subjects produced only an average of less than 8 animal names.

Discussion

This study provides some support to the postulate that optimal performance in a word-naming task is indeed related to the identification of the greatest number of semantic subfields and to the maximal production of items for each of these subfields. Given this verification, Study III gives some idea of the behavior associated with the lowered word-naming performance of RBD subjects. It appears that the smaller number of items produced by RBD subjects is associated with the fact that these subjects both identify a smaller number of semantic subfields *and* exploit each of these subfields less efficiently, at least for those subfields for which subjects tend to be the most productive.

These results show that RBD subjects are not impaired in their use of the appropriate strategy necessary to perform a word-naming task. Indeed, even though both strategies used are less efficient for RBD than for C subjects, RBD subjects still identify a certain number of subfields and still exploit them, at least to a certain degree. Indeed, if RBD subjects had had a problem using the appropriate strategy when confronted with the word-naming task, it would probably have manifested itself either (a) as a deficiency in the identification of different semantic subfields but with an intact exploitation of each subfield, (b) as an impairment in the exploitation of each subfield with respect to a normal number of different subfields produced, or even (c) as an absence of strategy, that is, producing unrelated words, each of which being nonetheless linked to the superordinate. In other words, RBD subjects' lowered word-naming performance does not appear to be due to the absence of one or the other of the strategies used by C subjects in order to perform such a task, rather, results show that it is the application of these strategies which is less efficient in RBD subjects.

These results emphasize the existence of a problem in the semantic organization itself or in the access to it more than a problem with the strategies used by a subject to perform in a given task. The fact that the total number of different items produced by the 20 C subjects is significantly larger than that produced by all 30 RBD subjects could indicate that RBD-subjects suffer a restriction of their functional semantic fields. It remains to be determined, however, whether the reduced efficiency of those two task-constrained strategies is specific to the postinitial moment of the task or if it is present throughout the task. Given the results of Study II, it could logically be hypothesized that the situations noted here, i.e., smaller number of subfields identified and reduced exploitation of each subfield, are probably present only after the postinitial period and thus account for the reduced word-naming performance during that phase of the task when response is less automatic.

The lowered word-naming performance of RBD subjects that following from Study II, was attributed to a problem in those less automatic processes necessary for lexical scan rather than to a gross problem in semantic organization could have two meanings. First it could mean that item-to-item semantic activation is somewhat less efficient in RBD subjects, thus restricting the number of different subfields as well as the number of different items. It could also mean that the processes permitting access to semantic organization are less efficent. Even though the present results do not identify which of these two problems is reponsible for lowered RBD subjects' performance, combined results of Studies II and III suggest that the problem may be one of semantic activation or one of access. It could be that this is true only when activation and/or access is dependent on or integrated in less automatic or more controlled processes. Further studies are needed in order to evaluate this hypothesis.

General Discussion

The studies reported here allow us to answer some, though not all, of the questions that were posed in the introduction. Results of the first two studies clearly indicate that the occurrence of a right-brain lesion does impair performance when subjects are given a lexicosemantic task requiring not only reference to semantic knowledge but also active production of lexical items. Moreover, it can be concluded that such an impairment is not the result of some nonspecific factor since (a) it is criterion-specific, (b) it is not accompanied either by a general increase of errors or by a modification of error type patterns, and (c) it is not apparent at the onset of the task. Results of the third study, interpreted in the context of those of the second study, reveal further that RBD subjects' production is not only quantitatively, but also qualitatively different from that of control subjects. It is suggested that the main problem with RBD subjects lies in their less automatic – or controlled – activation and/or access of the semantic component of the lexicon. This expresses itself as a specific reduction of word-naming performance after the initial moment of such a task, the latter depending upon the integrity of more automatic use of the same processes. Our results do not indicate that the possible contribution of the right hemisphere to semantic activation is exclusive to that hemisphere, nor would we like to advance such an hypothesis. In fact, our results could indicate that this contribution is not necessarily *specific* to the right hemisphere. It could be hypothesized that left-brain-damaged nonaphasic subjects would also exhibit lowered word-naming performance for semantic criteria that could be due to the same impairment in conscious activation of the lexicon. If this is the case, any task requiring conscious lexical retrieval on the basis of semantic criteria would be affected by a lesion of either hemisphere.

The results from a brain-damaged population are compatible with those of studies of the same processes in normal subjects. For instance, Chiarello (1985, this volume) has reported that automatic semantic priming – dependent automatic activation of the lexicon – is efficient in both hemifields, whereas controlled priming – dependent on the conscious activation of the lexicon – is more efficient in the right visual hemifield (left hemisphere). Thus, the first part of Chiarello's observation explains why automatic activation is not affected in RBD subjects, since it is proposed that the left hemisphere is also capable of this type of activation. However, the second part of chiarello's observation, and the fact that a lesion of the right hemisphere manifests itself more as a problem with controlled activation (and/or access) of the lexicon, permit one to hypothesize that even if the left hemisphere demonstrates the greatest potential for controlled semantic processes, these processes are *not* restricted to this hemisphere. This means that optimal controlled or conscious semantic processing requires the normal function of the right hemisphere.

Results of the present study also bring up the question of specificity of the right hemisphere's contribution to lexical semantics, and further, specificity of the contribution of those processes we referred to with regard to language itself. Studies like those we have been considering surely indicate that the integrity of the right hemisphere appears important for proper lexicosemantic function, mostly for its proper semantic aspects. This is claimed despite the fact that some reservations can be mentioned vis-à-vis the recourse to a group of subjects with CVA (Bogen 1985). In fact, the present results are not the only ones which suggest this and thus converging evidences exist. In contrast, it may be that these processes are not exclusive to language, as is semantic organization itself; it remains true, however, that they are certainly necessary for the efficiency of lexicosemantic processing. Not only does the right hemisphere show some semantic potential, as shown by numerous studies reviewed earlier, but it is claimed here that the integrity of the right hemisphere is necessary in order to actively use this semantic knowledge in the context of language production. However, it is not possible to identify here those specific aspects of lexical semantics or those particular lexicosemantic processes which are affected following a right-hemisphere lesion more than to say that the problem lies in the grey zone of semantics consisting of lexical access processes and/or semantic representations. Additional studies are needed to further elucidate the exact nature of the right hemisphere's contribution to lexical semantics and its relation with that of the left hemisphere.

Acknowledgements. Yves Joanette is scholar of the *Conseil de recherches médicales du Canada.* The authors wish to thank François Dehaut for the data analyses and Louise Bourret for the illustrations, as well as John Boeglin and John Ryalls for reviewing the manuscript.

References

Beaumont JG (1982) Studies with verbal stimuli. In: Beaumont JG (ed) Divided visual field studies of cerebral organisation. Academic, New York, pp 58–86

Benton AL (1968) Differential behavioral effects in frontal lobe disease. Neuropsychologia 6:53–60

Bogen JE (1985) The dual brain: some historical and methodological aspects. In: Benson DF, Zaidel E (eds) The dual brain. Guilford, New York, pp 27–43

Boller F (1968) Latent aphasias: right and left "nonaphasic" brain-damaged patients compared. Cortex 4:245–256

Bolter JF, Long CJ, Wagner M (1983) The utility of the Thurstone word fluency test in identifying cortical damage. J Clin Neuropsychol 5:77–82

Borkowski JG, Benton AL, Spreen O (1967) Word fluency and brain damage. Neuropsychologia 5:135–140

Bradshaw JL, Nettleton NC (1983) Human cerebral laterality. Prentice-Hall, Englewood Cliffs

Bradshaw JL, Gates A, Nettleton NC (1977) Bihemispheric involvement in lexical decision: handedness and a possible sex difference. Neuropsychologia 14:129–133

Bruyer R, Tuyumbu B (1980) Fluence verbale et lésion du cortex cérébral: performances et types d'erreurs. Encéphale 6:287–297

Chiarello C (1985) Hemisphere dynamics in lexical access: automatic and controlled priming. Brain Lang 26:146–172

Coltheart M (1980) Deep dyslexia: a right hemisphere hypothesis. In: Coltheart M, Patterson K, Marshall J (eds) Deep dyslexia. Routledge and Kegan Paul, London, pp 326–380

Gainotti G, Caltagirone C, Miceli G (1983) Selective impairment of semantic-lexical discrimination in right-brain-damaged patients. In: Perecman E (ed) Cognitive processing in the right hemisphere. Academic, New York, pp 149–168

Gazzaniga MS (1983) Right hemisphere language following brain bisection. A 20-year perspective. Am Psychol 38:525–537

Gazzaniga MS, Hillyard SA (1978) Language and speech capacity of the right hemisphere. Neuropsychologia 9:273–280

Gazzaniga MS, Sperry RW (1967) Language after section of the cerebral commissures. Brain 90:131–148

Goulet P, Joanette Y (in preparation) Semantic clustering in right-brain-damaged righthanders

Grossman M (1981) A bird is a bird is a bird: making reference within and without superordinate categories. Brain Lang 12:313–331

Hannequin D, Goulet P, Joanette Y (1987) La contribution de l'hémisphère droit à la communication verbale. Masson, Paris

Hécaen H, Albert M (1978) Human neuropsychology. Wiley, New York

Joanette Y, Goulet P (1986) Criterion-specific reduction of verbal fluency in right brain-damaged right-handers. Neuropsychologia 24(6):875–879
Joanette Y, Goulet P, Le Dorze G (1988) Impaired word-naming in right brain-damaged right-handers. Brain Lang 34(1):54–64
Lesser R (1974) Verbal comprehension in aphasia: an English version of three Italian tests. Cortex 10:247–263
Marcie P, Hécaen H, Dubois J, Angelergues R (1965) Les troubles de la réalisation de la parole au cours des lésions de l'hemisphère droit. Neuropsychologia 3:217–247
Millar JM, Whitaker HA (1983) The right hemisphere's contribution to language: a review of the evidence from brain-damaged subjects. In: Segalowitz S (ed) Language functions and brain organization. Academic, New York, pp 87–113
Milner B (1964) Some effects of frontal lobectomy in man. In: Warren JM, Akert K (eds) The frontal granular cortex and behavior. McGraw-Hill, New York, pp 313–331
Ober BA, Dronkers NF, Koss E, Delis DC, Friedland RP (1986) Retrieval from semantic memory in Alzheimer-type dementia. J Clin Exp Neuropsychol 8:75–92
Oldfield OD (1971) The assessment and analysis of handedness: the Edinburgh Inventory. Neuropsychologia 9:97–113
Perret E (1974) The left frontal lobe of man and the suppression of habitual responses in verbal categorical behaviour. Neuropsychologia 12:323–330
Ramier A, Hécaen H (1970) Rôle respectif des atteintes frontales et de la latéralisation lésionnelle dans les déficits de la «fluence verbale». Rev Neurol (Paris) 123:17–22
Rosen WG (1980) Verbal fluency in aging and dementia. J Clin Neuropsychol 2:135–146
Saffran EM, Bogyo LC, Schwartz M, Marin O (1980) Does deep dyslexia reflect right-hemisphere reading? In: Coltheart M, Patterson K, Marshall J (eds) Deep dyslexia. Routledge and Kegan Paul, London, pp 381–406
Searleman A (1983) Language capabilities of the right hemisphere. In: Young AW (ed) Functions of the right cerebral hemisphere. Academic, New York, pp 87–111
Thurstone L (1938) Primary mental abilities. University of Chicago Press, Chicago
Winer BJ (1971) Statistical principles in experimental design. McGraw-Hill, New York
Zaidel E (1983) A response to Gazzaniga. Language in the right hemisphere, convergent perspectives. Am Psychol 38:542–546

Appreciation of Metaphoric and Connotative Word Meaning by Brain-Damaged Patients *

HIRAM H. BROWNELL

Introduction

Language is often discussed in terms of separate parts, including the phonological, syntactic, and lexical components of the grammar. These components differ with respect to their connections to other domains of cognition. Unlike the other components, the lexicon, which contains a speaker's knowledge of individual words, represents a bridge between world knowledge and the language system. Words in the lexicon are linked to associated meanings that include a wealth of information about the world and that pertain to virtually all realms of a person's experience. In what follows, the term *lexical semantics* will be used to refer to the lexicon plus the range of associations that are often excluded from the lexicon proper (e.g., Emmorey and Fromkin, in press).

This chapter reviews some contributions of the two cerebral hemispheres to lexical-semantic ability. Over a century of work in aphasia and decades of work in laterality research (using neurologically intact subjects) have confirmed the major role of the left hemisphere in lexical semantics (see Chiarello, in press, and Lesser 1978, for reviews). What is argued in this and other chapters in this volume is that the right hemisphere also makes important contributions in this domain.

For the most part, the work to be discussed in this chapter describes the lexical-semantic deficits of patients who have suffered unilateral brain damage due to stroke. Every research methodology has its advantages and disadvantages, but some features of using neurological populations deserve special mention. When one observes a selective deficit in a patient with focal brain disease, the usual inference is that the damaged region is somehow involved in mediating that performance in a neurologically intact person. It is important to note that such deficits arise despite the ability of noninvolved regions to compensate, i.e., to take over the functions usually performed by the damaged area. Thus, deficits observed subsequent to focal brain injury represent conservative estimates of the abilities that a damaged region is normally involved in since the observed deficits reflect those functions that other regions are not able to take over.

* The preparation of this chapter was supported by NIH grants NS11408 and 06209 and by the Research Service of the Veterans Administration.

This chapter reviews work bearing on two related aspects of lexical semantics: appreciation of metaphoric and of connotative word meanings. First, the topics of metaphor comprehension and the distinction between denotative and connotative meaning will be introduced in the context of work carried out with neurologically intact subject populations. Then, results of research with brain-damaged patients that bear on these two areas will be reviewed, with particular attention paid to the role of the right hemisphere. Finally, some implications of the neuropsychological data will be discussed.

Metaphoric and Connotative Meaning

One broad distinction in meaning is that between a word's denotation and connotation or, equivalently, between its cognitive and emotive meaning (Lyons 1968; Palmer 1976). Denotation specifies a concept's literal meaning, i.e., its "dictionary" meaning. For example, "capitalism" refers to an economic system whose features include private ownership and a profit motive, and "communism" refers to a system whose features include public ownership of means of production. In contrast to a term's denotation, its connotation specifies more associative aspects of its meaning. For most speakers of American English the concept of capitalism carries a generally positive association while communism carries a negative connotation. There will be some variation in how different speakers of the same language code the connotation of some terms. A conservative Republican may have a more negative view of communism that do members of the American Communist Party. However, most speakers in a culture will code similar connotations – as well as similar denotations – for concepts, thereby insuring accurate communication.

As suggested above, the primary quality of connotation is its emotive value, such as whether a term signifies a generally positive (e.g., birth) or negative (e.g., death) concept. This emotive component often seems extrinsic to the precise, dictionary meaning of the term; however, full appreciation of this type of semantic information is necessary to a language user to completely understand word meanings in all their richness. The caustic, demeaning, or insulting quality of many derogatory terms (e.g., spinster, slumlord) and the positive meaning of complimentary terms (e.g., saint) are carried by their connotations. In addition, sensitivity to connotation helps a speaker to apprehend and exploit metaphoric correspondences between concepts that are denotatively unrelated.

A second salient difference between denotative and connotative meaning components is their generality of application. Denotative attributes for the most part are highly specific in that they distinguish concepts in one semantic domain but do not apply across other domains. For example, the differences between types of economic systems (e.g., capitalism versus communism) do not figure in the distinctions between types of vehicles (car versus airplane), or between types of cars (sedan versus convertible). While there are some very general denotative distinctions, e.g., human versus nonhuman, connotative attributes, in contrast, routinely figure in concepts from highly disparate domains. For example, the positive versus negative connotative distinction applied here to economic systems applies equally to concepts in domains as different as foods (steak versus creamed chipped beef) and professions (statesman versus politician). In this sense, components of connotative meaning are typically much more general in their applicability than are most denotative semantic components.

There is disagreement about the relevance of connotative meaning to the lexicon (see, e.g., Clark and Clark 1977). One point of opposition is the distinction between dictionary and encyclopedia views on what knowledge ought to be included in the lexicon. According to the dictionary view, the contents of a word's representation in the lexicon proper should be limited to the syntactic and denotative information needed to define the word and its role in sentence processing. On this view, general associations are be stored in some (extralinguistic) auxiliary memory. According to the encyclopedia view, this range of associations would form an integral part of a word's lexical representation. Thus for communism, the associations for an American English speaker might include a generally negative connotation, a strong link to the Soviet Union, and restrictions on freedom of expression. These and similar associations would not be stored in the lexicon according to a strict dictionary view of the lexicon, but they would be included on a broader, encyclopedia view.

Quite apart from whether or not connotation forms part of a word's lexical entry, there is considerable empirical work that establishes the psychological reality of connotation and confirms its major role in lexical-semantic processing. Osgood et al. (1957) were able to extract the connotations of a large body of common English nouns drawn from a number of very different semantic domains. These authors asked subjects to judge each word's relative value on a number of semantic scales identified using word pairs such as happy-sad and hard-soft. The ratings were then analyzed (using factor analysis) to abstract out the common dimensions that reflected subjects' perceived similarities among all the rated words. They were able to identify three general connotative factors or dimensions of meaning – evaluation (good, bad), potency (strength), and activity – along which each word could be assigned a value, regardless of its denotative meaning. These three semantic dimensions, by virtue of the analytic techniques used on the data, collapsed across different semantic domains and, thus, represented general kinds of semantic information that subjects had stored as part of their knowledge of word meanings.

More recent work in cognitive psychology has used a related analytic technique (multidimensional scaling) to reveal the semantic dimensions that capture psychologically real differences among animal concepts in semantic memory (e.g., Caramazza et al. 1976; Rips et al. 1973). Specifically, subjects were asked to judge the similarity between all possible pairs constructed from a set of animal concepts (e.g., lion-dog, lion-hawk, dog-hawk). These similarity judgments were then analyzed to extract a small set of dimensions that accounted for subjects' between-concept similarity judgments. Subjects in these studies typically rated stimuli as similar on the basis of denotative distinctions such as species membership (e.g., all else being equal, fish were judged as similar to other fish and relatively dissimilar to birds). However, subjects also made distinctions based on connotative notions such as ferocity. A hawk, for example, was judged as similar to a shark because both are fierce.

In addition to playing a role in subjects' judgments of semantic similarity, connotative semantic content helps predict how easily subjects can verify a stimulus' membership in a superordinate category such as "bird" (Rips et al. 1973). For example, the category "bird" has a prototypical value along several semantic dimensions, including the connotative dimension of ferocity. These prototypical values are approximated by the average value on each dimension of all the members of the category (cf., Rosch et al. 1976). On average, subjects will verify category membership more quickly (more easily) for members having, for example, a degree of ferocity approximately equal to the category's prototypical value on that dimension (McCloskey and Glucksberg 1979; Smith et al. 1974).

Metaphor appreciation constitutes another realm in which aspects of meaning that can be applied in different semantic domains play a major role. The ubiquity and communicative effectiveness of metaphor and its role in the growth of a language's lexicon are uncontroversial. The "mouth" of a river, the "eye" of a needle, and the "leg" of a table represent extensions of literal meanings tied to parts of the body, just as "skyscraper" and "software" illustrate how new concepts can be expressed by a metaphoric application of existing words. Brown (1958) has described the basis for metaphoric extension of concepts such as warm, cold, and dull. Indeed, it is often difficult to draw a precise distinction between metaphoric extension of a concept's meaning and nonmetaphoric polysemy (see, e.g., Miller 1979, for discussion of these points).

The hallmark of metaphor is the use of semantic information that can be applied across semantic domains and that, sometimes, depends on connotative similarity for effectiveness. One familiar example discussed by Ortony et al. (1978) is "billboards are warts on the landscape." The topic of the metaphor (billboards) is linked to the vehicle (warts) by the ground of the ugliness attributed to an unwanted protrusion on a surface. Intuitively, the impact of the metaphor is in part attributable to the strength of the negative associations of warts, and in part to the fact that both warts and billboards protrude from the skin and the landscape, respectively. The extreme differences between the denotations of warts and billboards serve to accentuate those connotative similarities that exist independently of the concepts' respective semantic domains. Certainly not all metaphors depend on strong positive or negative connotations for their effectiveness, but many do, and all metaphors rest on some application of information from one domain in another.

While much of the psychological literature on metaphor comprehension centers on topics such as the role of similarity and analogy (e.g., Ortony 1979), Glucksberg et al. (1982) offer a different perspective. They argue that processing metaphoric potential is mandatory, i.e., that a listener cannot help but assess whether a combination of words, whose literal meanings are incompatible, can be interpreted metaphorically. In a series of studies, Glucksberg et al. used a variant of the Stroop interference paradigm (1935). Subjects were timed as they judged the literal truth of sentences. The critical stimulus items included two kinds of literally false sentences: those with (Some jobs are prisons.) and those without (Some jobs are birds.) metaphoric potential. Subjects took longer to reject the literal truth of those sentences with metaphoric interpretations: Even when doing so hurt their performances, subjects could not ignore the metaphors. In light of these results, Glucksberg et al. suggest that the mental processes used to automatically evaluate metaphors are the same as those used to evaluate sentences' literal meanings. The implication is that normal subjects' basic language abilities support a facility with metaphor comprehension, or at least awareness of metaphoric potential regardless of whether such awareness is acted upon. Accordingly, disrupted processing of metaphors may provide a means of examining components of language performance.

Neuropsychological Evidence

There have been several investigations of how metaphor appreciation can be affected by brain disease. In a well-known study, Winner and Gardner (1977) examined the abilities of unilaterally left- and right-brain-damaged patients to understand familiar phrasal metaphors such as "He has a heavy heart." Subjects were read a phrase and then asked to select the corresponding picture from a set of four alternatives. The alternatives included (1) a depiction of the correct, metaphoric meaning, e.g., a man crying, (2) a literal foil, e.g., a man straining to carry an oversized heart, (3) a representation of the noun used in the metaphor, e.g., a picture of just a heart, and (4) a representation of the adjective used in the metaphor, e.g., a picture of a lead weight.

The right-hemisphere-damaged (RHD) patients made many errors on this task relative to (non-brain-damaged) normal control subjects. More specifically, the RHD patients tended to choose the literal foil approximately as often as the correct, metaphoric response. In contrast, the left-hemisphere-damaged (LHD) patients (all of whom were aphasic) scored slightly better than the RHD patients and were much less attracted to the literal foils. The LHD patients performed more "normally" despite their language disturbances. Not only were the LHD patients not especially attracted to the literal foils, they often laughed at them. This basic result of an excessive literalness affecting RHD patients' comprehension of language materials has been confirmed and extended by several authors (Kempler et al. 1984; Myers and Linebaugh 1981; Stachowiak et al. 1977).

This tendency towards a literal interpretation of phrasal stimuli is striking. One reason is the highly familiar nature of the items used: Right-hemisphere damage is traditionally thought not to greatly affect old linguistic knowledge (i.e., knowledge of word meanings and syntactic rules acquired before the onset of illness). In addition, the preferred reading for these items is metaphoric: The effect of right-sided damage was to bias subjects towards the less likely, literal interpretations. The direction of this effect runs counter to the usual pattern that brain damage impairs appreciation of low frequency items more than appreciation of high frequency items (Lesser 1978).

The effects of right-hemisphere brain damage on appreciation of denotation and connotation has received less attention in the neuropsychological literature, although some relevant issues have been addressed. Zurif et al. (1974), for example, used a set of animal and human terms to ascertain the effects of left-hemisphere brain damage on aphasic patients' use of species membership, a denotative distinction, as opposed to degree of ferocity a connotative distinction, in a similarity judgment task. The most relevant part of the stimulus set consisted of the following concepts: shark, trout, turtle, and crocodile. These concepts could be distinguished on the basis of species membership: trout and shark are similar in this respect; or on the basis of ferocity: trout and turtle are similar in this respect. The results revealed that the normal control subjects in this study focused on species membership as a basis for judging similarity while aphasic patients with left anterior brain damage instead focused on ferocity. Because no patients with unilateral right-sided brain damage were tested, this study does not speak to the contribution of the right hemisphere, but the results obtained show how use of some types of connotative information may be preserved while use of some denotative information is curtailed.

Gardner and Denes (1973) have reported some preliminary data on RHD patients' appreciation of connotation. Based on work by Osgood (1960), Gardner and Denes used a pictorial adaptation of the semantic differential (Osgood et al. 1957). Gardner and Denes' task involved matching a concept such as wealth or poverty with a nonrepresentational line drawing. On each trial, a subject was presented with a concept and asked to choose which of two line drawings the concept went with best. The drawings were designed to capture an aspect of a term's connotation. For example, for the concept wealth, a subject might have to choose between a set of arrows pointing up and a set of arrows pointing down. The canonical response which was chosen for each item by at least 80% of a group of normal pilot subjects was the set of arrows pointing up, presumably reflecting the generally positive connotation of wealth. LHD patients in this task performed worse than the normal control subjects, but more interesting was that the authors also attempted testing with a small group of six RHD patients. Some of these RHD patients either could not or would not do the task, and all of them took issue with the task requirements. The three RHD patients who completed the task peformed roughly at the level of the LHD patients, although no statistical comparison was reported.

A more recent study (Brownell et al. 1984) used purely verbal stimuli to more directly compare the effects of unilateral left- and right-hemisphere brain damage on patients' sensitivity to connotative and denotative meaning, and, in addition, on patients' sensitivity to a form of metaphoric equivalence. The stimuli were assembled from a set of eight dimensional adjectives: warm, cold, deep, shallow, loving, hateful, wise, and foolish. This particular set of adjective concepts was chosen because its members could be used to represent a variety of relevant semantic relations or types of semantic relatedness. For example, the concepts warm, deep, loving, and wise all share a positive connotation, while cold, shallow, hateful, and foolish share a negative connotation.

In addition to a general connotative similarity, certain of these adjectives share a more specific link that rests on what can be termed metaphoric equivalence (e.g., Brown 1958). For example, the dominant, more frequent meaning of warm refers to temperature, but the word also has an alternative meaning – affectionate – in the very different semantic domain of personality traits. The words warm and loving thus share an equivalence beyond shared polarity that perhaps stems from the comfort and warmth of a hug and the comfort and security of a friendship. Similarly, cold and hateful share a metaphoric equivalence, as do deep and wise, and shallow and foolish.

These adjective concepts can also be equated according to other criteria that are more closely tied to denotative meaning. One general distinction made is that between human and nonhuman terms (e.g., Keil 1979). Terms (loving, hateful, wise, foolish) whose dominant meanings concern personality descriptions can be separated from those terms (warm, cold, deep, shallow) whose dominant meanings apply to physical characteristics. A more specific type of denotative semantic relation is antonymy: wise–foolish, deep–shallow, etc. Clark (1970), for example, explored the psychological implications of the near equivalence between a dimensional adjective and its antonym, i.e., that they have the same semantic composition except for the one critical component specifying polarity.

The empirical question asked in the Brownell et al. study was whether right-hemisphere brain damage selectively curtailed patients' use of either connotative or metaphoric word meaning. To test for such highly selective deficits, a semantic judgment task was designed to reveal which types of semantic relations subjects would use as a basis for responding. Subjects were presented with all possible word triplets constructed from the eight adjectives and were asked to select the two that were the most related, i.e., that went together best. Each word in the set of eight could be related to the others in several different ways. As an illustration, consider the word triplet warm–loving–cold. A subject might decide that warm and cold are the most related on the basis of their antonymic relation. Alternatively, the subject might choose warm and loving on the basis of their metaphoric equivalence. Finally, the subject might have grouped loving and cold together. This final pairing would represent an error since there is no obvious semantic link between these two words. Analogously, with a different triplet, warm–wise–shallow, the subject might group warm and wise together on the basis of a shared positive connotation; or he or she might choose warm and shallow since these two apply most frequently to the physical domain while wise refers to a personality trait.

In this study, groups of unilaterally LHD and RHD patients and normal control subjects were tested. The data were analyzed using a hierarchical clustering program (Hartigan 1981) to determine which types of semantic relatedness were used by subjects in the three groups. The clustering solution for the RHD patients showed that as a group they focused on denotative relations: RHD patients used antonymic relations most consistently and also grouped words by shared domain of applicability, i.e., whether a term applied primarily to humans (personality traits) or to physical objects. They showed no clear use of either metaphoric or connotative relatedness. In marked contrast, the LHD patients' solution revealed a general grouping of words by shared connotation and a strong sensitivity to metaphoric equivalence beyond what could be attributed to connotative similarity alone. The LHD patients' solution did not show any consistent use of antonymy. The solution for the non-brain-damaged control subjects showed consistent use of both antonymy and metaphoric equivalence. It should be noted, though, that inferential statistical analysis revealed that the differences between the patient groups in their use of general connotative information, i.e., polarity, and in their use of domain of applicability were not as strong as the other effects and must therefore be interpreted more cautiously.

Two different accounts can be offered for these lexical-semantic deficits observed in RHD patients. The first is that the observed deficits are specific to metaphor and, perhaps, also to connotation. A second account is that RHD patients are rigid and therefore have trouble generating alternative readings for all linguistic stimuli. This rigidity could account for most of the deficits described above and also suggests a common explanation for RHD patients' impaired performances with alternative meanings of other linguistic units. For example, RHD patients show impaired appreciation of alternative readings of indirect requests (Foldi 1987, Hirst et al. 1984) and other potentially ambiguous sentences in context (Brownell et al. 1986).

A subsequent study (Brownell et al. submitted for publication) was designed to test whether the observed deficits were specific to metaphoric alternative meanings or were just one manifestation of a pervasive difficulty of RHD patients dealing with all instances of linguistic ambiguity. This new study compared subjects' appreciation of alternative meanings of two kinds of polysemous words, potentially metaphoric adjectives such as those used in the Brownell et al. (1984) study and nonmetaphoric polysemous nouns such as "cabinet" (meaning either a cupboard or a group of advisors). The reasoning was that a pervasive rigidity would affect both types of polysemous words equally, while a deficit specific to metaphor processing would be limited in scope.

The experimental task was based on word triads constructed as follows. Each triad consisted of an ambiguous target word (e.g., cabinet), a close synonym (advisors) of the target's secondary or less dominant meaning, and a nonsynonymous associate (dishes) of its dominant meaning. The study included two types of triads: those described above based on nonmetaphoric noun targets, and other triads based on potentially metaphoric adjective targets (e.g., warm), a close synonym of the target's secondary alternative meaning (loving), and an associate of the target's dominant meaning (blanket). In addition, both the metaphoric and nonmetaphoric triads varied in the degree of relatedness between a target's alternative meanings. In some triads the two meanings were quite close semantically (e.g., quick: fast, smart) while in other triads, the two meanings were less related (e.g., suit: garment, trial). Subjects in this study were then presented with these triads and asked to select the two words out of each triad that were most similar in meaning.

The task proved very easy for normal control subjects, who performed at ceiling levels. These data were not analyzed further since they yielded no information on the relative difficulty of retrieving and using both metaphoric and nonmetaphoric alternative meanings. This near perfect performance was to be expected on the basis of earlier work showing that control subjects were sensitive to the metaphoric alternative meanings of adjectives (Brownell et al. 1984) and that in general normal subjects have easy access to words' alternative meanings (see Simpson 1984, for a review). Similarly, a small proportion (3 out of 18) of RHD patients tested also performed at ceiling, and their data were discarded.

Of greatest interest here is the specificity of the RHD patients' lexical-semantic deficit. The relevant comparison is between the RHD patients' performances on the two types of triads and the performances of LHD patients. The LHD patients in this study performed equally well on the metaphoric and the nonmetaphoric triads, while the RHD patients performed significantly worse on the metaphoric triads, that is, the RHD patients were especially drawn to the nonsynonymous associates of the metaphoric adjectives' literal meanings. Relative to the LHD patients, the RHD patients showed a selective deficit for the appreciation of metaphoric alternative word meanings.

One other difference between the patient groups suggests that the two groups processed the metaphoric triads differently. The LHD patients, but not the RHD patients, showed a significant effect of the relatedness between the metaphoric targets' alternative meanings. The LHD patients performed better when the alternative meanings of a target were closer semantically than when they were less related, but the RHD patients showed no such effect. (Neither patient group showed a relatedness effect for the nonmetaphoric noun triads.)

A final comparison performed using these data argues against a purely affective factor as an explanation for the RHD patients' poor performances. This issue is important for understanding the nature of this lexical deficit since these patients routinely exhibit deficits in processing affective material (Etcoff

1985; Heilman et al. 1985; Tucker 1981). The metaphoric adjective trials were divided into more- and less-affective sets on the basis of pilot subject ratings, but when the RHD patients' performances on the two sets were compared, no difference was found.

In all, these results suggest that the RHD patients have a metaphor-specific lexical-semantic dysfunction and that they process metaphoric potential differently than do LHD patients. However, it should also be emphasized that most of the patients tested were also clearly impaired relative to normal control subjects in their appreciation of nonmetaphoric, as well as metaphoric, alternative meanings. This last result is consistent with a pervasive deficit in appreciation of alternative meanings. RHD patients may simply exhibit separate deficits, only one of which is specific to processing metaphor.

Summary and Implications

The effects of right-sided brain damage suggest several roles for the right hemisphere in normal lexical-semantic processing. One possibility has been proposed elsewhere (see Chiarello's chapter, this volume, and Burgess and Simpson 1988): The right hemisphere is involved in the maintenance of alternative meanings of ambiguous words and phrases encountered during language comprehension. These alternative readings are available initially to both hemispheres, but at later stages of processing the left hemisphere actively inhibits alternative meanings, which are thereafter available only to the right hemisphere. In a sense, the right hemisphere acts as a memory buffer that keeps unlikely readings available just in case they turn out to be relevant, such as when a listener's initial interpretation of a word or phrase ends up not fitting with a larger context. This view offers an explanation for why RHD patients seem consistently impaired whenever an initially unlikely alternative interpretation of a linguistic element must be retrieved and used during comprehension.

An attractive feature of this account is its generality. First, it offers a single explanation for RHD patients' comprehension deficits with a wide range of language materials ranging from the single word (e.g., Brownell et al. 1984) to whole utterances in context (e.g., Hirst et al. 1984). Second, this memorial account provides a theoretical structure for interpreting data drawn from studies of impaired subjects and from laterality studies performed with neurologically intact subjects (Chiarello et al. 1987; Burgess and Simpson 1988).

This putative memorial function, however, does not exhaust the likely contributions of the right hemisphere to lexical semantics. A difficulty processing alternative meanings cannot by itself explain RHD patients' problems with connotation. The Gardner and Denes (1973) study and the Brownell et al. (1984) study both revealed possible deficits that go beyond appreciation of either metaphoric or nonmetaphoric alternative meanings. While additional empirical confirmation of these effects is needed, the right hemisphere appears to play a significant role in the full appreciation of the emotive associations that form part of words' meanings. This connotation deficit may well figure in the general affective dysfunction that characterizes many of these patients. It is, though, important to note the specificity of this lexical affective impairment: RHD patients do not typically show marked difficulty with the denotative content of emotion words (Etcoff 1984). That the selective effects of unilateral brain damage reinforce the division between connotative and denotative meaning suggests a means of isolating specifically lexical processing from more general lexical-semantic ability. If successful, this avenue of neuropsychological research could define the boundary between the language system and general cognition.

Finally, RHD patients have trouble with metaphoric processing over and above what can be accounted for on the basis of a pervasive problem with alternative meanings or on the basis of an affective limitation. Thus, another possible role for the right hemisphere is specific to metaphoric processing, although the specific nature of this role is still not known. The right hemisphere may be critical for apprehending the extension of a term's meaning – or, more precisely, selected parts of a term's meaning – to a different domain, something which normal subjects do automatically (Glucksberg et al. 1982). Or, the right hemisphere may play a major part in responding appropriately on the basis of metaphoric equivalence once it has been understood. This latter alternative fits well with Glucksberg et al.'s suggestion that the same language processes are used to understand both literal and nonliteral language. Since RHD patients' basic language abilities are largely intact, perhaps their metaphor deficit is due to some postcomprehension processing abnormality. In any event, finer analyses of RHD patients' processing deficits will be needed to ascertain just how their metaphor appreciation goes awry and how this deficit interacts with other processes relevant to language use.

Acknowledgements. I thank Ray Molloy for his comments on an earlier draft, Nancy Lefkowitz, Director of Speech and Language Pathology, and other personnel of the Spaulding Rehabilitation Hospital for their support of much of the research described in this chapter.

References

Brown RW (1958) Words and things. Free Press Glencoe, IL

Brownell HH, Potter HH, Michelow D, Gardner G (1984) Sensitivity to lexical denotation and connotation in brain-damaged patients: a double dissociation? Brain Lang 22:253–265

Brownell HH, Potter HH, Bihrle AM, Gardner H (1986) Inference deficits in right brain-damaged patients. Brain Lang 21:310–321

Brownell HH, Simpson TL, Bihrle AM, Potter HH, Gardner H (submitted) Appreciation of metaphoric alternative word meanings by left and right brain-damaged patients

Burgess C, Simpson GB (1988) Cerebral hemispheric mechanisms in the retrieval of ambiguous word meanings. Brain Lang 33:86–103

Caramazza A, Hersh HM, Torgerson WS (1976) Subjective structures and operations in semantic memory. J Verb Learn Verb Behav 15:103–118
Chiarello C (in press) Lateralization of lexical processes in the normal brain: a review of visual half-field research. In: Whitaker HA (ed) Contemporary reviews in neuropsychology. Springer, Berlin Heidelberg New York
Chiarello C, Senehi J, Nuding S (1987) Semantic priming with abstract and concrete words: differential asymmetry may be postlexical. Brain Lang 31:43–60
Clark HH (1970) Word associations and linguistic theory. In: Lyons J (ed) New horizons in linguistics. Penguin, Baltimore, pp 271–286
Clark HH, Clark EV (1977) Psychology and language. Harcourt Brace Jovanovich, New York
Emmorey KD, Fromkin VA (in press) The mental lexicon. In: Newmeyer F (ed) Linguistics: the Cambridge survey, vol 4. Cambridge University Press, New York
Etcoff NL (1984) Perceptual and conceptual organization of facial emotions: hemispheric differences. Brain Cogn 3:385–412
Etcoff NL (1985) The neuropsychology of emotional expression. Massachusetts Institute of Technology Center for Cognitive Science Occasional Paper no 31
Foldi NS (1987) Appreciation of pragmatic interpretations of indirect commands: comparison of right and left brain-damaged patients. Brain Lang 31:88–108
Gardner H, Denes G (1973) Connotative judgements by aphasic patients on a pictorial adaptation of the semantic differential. Cortex 9:183–196
Glucksberg S, Gildea P, Bookin HB (1982) On understanding nonliteral speech: can people ignore metaphors? J Verb Lern Verb Behav 21:85–98
Hartigan J (1981) P1M cluster analysis of variables. In: Dixon WJ (chief ed) BMDP statistical software. University of California Press, Berkeley CA, pp 448–455
Heilman KM, Bowers D, Valenstein E (1985) Emotional disorders associated with neurological diseases. In: Heilman KM, Valenstein E (eds) Clinical neuropsychology. Oxford University Press, New York, pp 377–402
Hirst W, LeDoux J, Stein S (1984) Constraints on the processing of indirect speech acts: evidence from aphasiology. Brain Lang 23:26–33
Keil FC (1979) Semantic and conceptual development. Harvard University Press, Cambridge, MA
Kempler D, Van Lancker D, Hadler B (1984) Familiar phrase recognition in brain-damaged and demented adults. Academy of Aphasia, Santa Monica, CA
Lesser R (1978) Psycholinguistic investigations of aphasia. Elsevier, New York
Lyons J (1968) Introduction to theoretical linguistics. Cambridge University Press, Cambridge
McCloskey M, Glucksberg S (1979) Decision processes in verifying membership statements: implications for models of semantic memory. Cogn Psychol 11:1–37
Miller GA (1979) Images and models, similes and metaphors. In: Ortony A (ed) Metaphor and thought. Cambridge University Press, New York, pp 202–250
Myers PS, Linebaugh CW (1981) Comprehension of idiomatic expressions by right-hemisphere-damaged adults. In: Brookshire RH (ed) Clinical aphasiology: conference proceedings. BRK, Minneapolis, pp 254–261
Ortony A (ed) (1979) Metaphor and thought. Cambridge University Press, New York
Ortony A, Reynolds RE, Arter JR (1978) Metaphor: theoretical and empirical research. Psychol Bull 85:919–943
Osgood CE (1960) The cross-cultural generality of visual-verbal synesthetic tendencies. Behav Sci 5:146–169
Osgood CE, Suci GJ, Tannenbaum PH (1957) The measurement of meaning. University of Illinois Press, Urbana, IL
Palmer FR (1976) Semantics. Cambridge University Press, New York
Rips LJ, Shoben EJ, Smith EE (1973) Semantic distance and the verification of semantic relations. J Verb Lern Verb Behav 12:1–20

Rosch E, Simpson C, Miller RS (1976) Structural bases of typicality effects. J Exp Psychol [Hum Percept] 2:491–502
Simpson GB (1984) Lexical ambiguity and its role in models of word recognition. Psychol Bull 96:316–340
Smith EE, Shoben EJ, Rips LJ (1974) Structure and process in semantic memory: a model for semantic decisions. Psychol Rev 81:214–241
Stachowiak FJ, Huber W, Poeck K, Kerschensteiner M (1977) Text comprehension in aphasia. Brain Lang 4:177–195
Stroop JR (1935) Studies of interference in serial verbal reactions. J Exp Psychol 18:643–662
Tucker DM (1981) Lateral brain function, emotion, and conceptualization. Psychol Bull 89:19–46
Winner E, Gardner H (1977) The comprehension of metaphor in brain-damaged patients. Brain 100:719–727
Zurif EB, Caramazza A, Myerson R, Galvin J (1974) Semantic feature representations for normal and aphasic language. Brain Lang 1:167–187

The Right Hemisphere's Access to Lexical Meaning: A Function of its Release from Left-Hemisphere Control? *

THEODOR LANDIS and MARIANNE REGARD

Introduction

Over a century ago Wigan (1844) stated: "That, in the healthy brain, one of the cerebra is almost always superior in power to the other, and capable of exercising control over the volitions of its fellow, and of preventing them from passing into acts, or from being manifested to others." The discrepancy between a sometimes astonishing language competence of the isolated right hemisphere in split-brain patients (for review see Zaidel 1985), or in adult hemispherectomy patients (Smith 1966), and the sometimes complete lack of language competence in aphasic patients despite an intact right hemisphere has led to a revival of the old idea that the dominant, controlling hemisphere inhibits the potential function of its opposite fellow (Moscovitch 1976; Landis et al. 1983; Regard et al. 1985; Zaidel 1985; Regard et al. 1986).

According to this view, reading, the process of gathering meaning from written information, which is commonly associated with left-hemisphere dominance, should have a hidden counterpart in the right hemisphere. Although both hemispheres are potentially able to read, they may weight lexical meaning differently, arrive at meaning via different paths of information processing, and may be attracted by different attributes of the same written information. We know that the two hemispheres' appreciation of lexical meaning dissociate with respect to concreteness and imageability of nouns (e.g., Ellis and Shepherd 1974; Day 1977; Richardson 1975). We have shown that this extends also to the emotional content of written words (Graves et al. 1981). When normal subjects perform lexical decisions on high-emotional versus low-emotional nouns (e.g., love and fact) they will detect both word classes better when presented to the left hemisphere than to the right hemisphere (without a significant distinction between the two word classes); but when presented to the right hemisphere, only high-emotional words are detected; the low-emotional words are not recognized as real words. This result suggests that depending on the hemisphere stimulated, two different reading processes are at work, one, the right hemispheric, being especially sensitive to the emotional aspect of the lexical meaning of words.

* This work has been supported by the Swiss National Science Foundation Grant Nr. 3.884.0.83 and has been presented in part at the EBBS Workshop on clinical neuropsychology, Zurich, April 1985, and at the 15th Meeting of the INS in Washington, February, 1987.

That the two hemispheres, in their attempt to derive meaning from written information, are attracted by very different aspects of the same stimulus is further exemplified by our recent observation of a double dissociation between the processing of written information and side of lesion (Landis and Regard 1988). The two patients concerned had ischemic posterior cerebral artery infarcts in opposite hemispheres. Whereas the patient with the left-sided lesion had pure alexia, the patient with the right-sided lesion had prosopagnosia (for clinical details see Campbell et al. 1986). Both patients recognized handwriting as written information. The patient with pure alexia, while not able to say *what* had been written, could nevertheless tell by *whom* it had been written through recognition of the handwriting. On the other hand, the patient with prosopagnosia recognized *what* had been written but not *who* had written it and complained of having lost the sense of familiarity of handwriting, including her own. These two patients with complementary posterior lesions, therefore, dissociated completely with respect to familiarity and verbal content of the same visual information. We therefore conjecture that familiarity and ability to verbalize may be regarded as two opposite gradients of dominance with respect to the hemisphere involved in decoding written information. According to the initial hypothesis, the left posterior hemisphere would control the opposite posterior brain for verbalization ability and vice versa for familiarity. Therefore, complete disconnection of the two posterior hemispheres or complete abolition of the left posterior hemisphere's function should improve the isolated right hemisphere's access to lexical meaning.

Right-Hemisphere Reading: Pure Alexia

A condition in which right-hemisphere reading could be expected is the classical clinical "disconnection" syndrome of pure alexia, where the right visual cortex is anatomically disconnected from the left hemisphere language zones by a left inferomedial occipitotemporal and a splenial lesion (Dejerine 1892; Geschwind 1965; for review: Greenblatt 1977; Damasio and Damasio 1983). Clinically, however, only a few of these patients have shown some reading ability when tested with multiple choice word–object or object–word matching or with matching of spoken names to a written word (Kreindler and Ionasescu 1961; Caplan and Hedley-Whyte 1974; Stachowiak and Poeck 1976; Assal and Regli 1980). Purely alexic patients did not, as would be theoretically predicted, behave like some split-brain patients (Benson and Geschwind 1969; Benson 1985) who can retrieve an object with the left hand which corresponds to an object name flashed in the left visual field, although they are unable to read the word and are verbally unaware of its presence (Zaidel 1978; Sperry et al. 1969).

A few years ago, however, we presented a purely alexic patient who did show the expected split-brain-like performance under special conditions (Landis et al. 1980). This patient, a typical letter-by-letter reader with a complete right homonymous hemianopia, was tested tachistoscopically subsequent to the removal of a left occipitotemporal glioblastoma. He was asked to fixate a central dot and stimuli were flashed in his left visual field (LVF), which projects to the healthy right hemisphere. Only at exposure durations which allowed for letter-by-letter reading, generally well above 1000 ms, was he able to read whole words of four and five letters. In order to read single letters he needed exposure durations of 50 ms. When presented with eight names of familiar objects at 30 ms, below the exposure he needed to recognize individual letters, he instantly read the first one correctly but for the remaining seven he said "I don't see anything, it is just a flash of light." From a display of 20 familiar objects (including an object sharing the same initial letter as each target word), we asked him to point "intuitively" to the objects whose names he had not been able to see or read aloud. To his own astonishment he pointed to the correct object in five of seven instances. This patient could extract meaning (shown by correct word–object matching) only at very short exposure durations, when he was verbally *unaware* of written information. In this condition stimulus presentation amounted to subliminal stimulation (for review see Dixon 1981; Holender 1986). Since the same unawareness of written information is the rule in split-brain patients, one may conjecture that verbal unawareness of lexical information may be the prerequisite for using the right hemisphere's reading capacity. Verbal awareness, even of minimal lexical information such as individual letters, would activate analytic, left-hemisphere reading, which in turn would inhibit right-hemisphere reading.

When we retested our patient later, his alexia was clinically unchanged, but he could then read single letters at exposures as short as 10 ms and was thus able to name some individual letters of words presented at 20 ms. When presented again with the eight names of familiar objects exposed for 20 ms, he instantly read two correctly, recognized individual letters in five of them, and denied having seen a word or even a single letter in the remaining one. However, only in the latter case could he point correctly to the corresponding object, while he mismatched the five words from which he was able to read individual letters.

This performance suggests that right-hemisphere reading is best or maybe exclusively demonstrated in a condition where verbal awareness is missing, that is, in a total functional disconnection from verbalization as is the case in split-brain patients. In our patient the *anatomical* disconnection was incomplete, since he was able to verbalize letters (letter-by-letter reading), but we suggest that the short exposure duration induced a complete *functional* disconnection. We conjecture that the presence of a significant degree of left-hemisphere (letter-by-letter), conscious verbal reading inhibits alternative right-hemisphere reading comprehension. As has been pointed out by Patterson and Kay (1982), Patterson and Besner (1984a, b), and more recently by Shallice and Saffran (1986), our theoretical speculations from this case are based on a limited number of observations. However, the correct choice of one object out of twenty is already a significant performance at the $P=0.05$ level. Five correct choices out of seven, as our patient produced, is a highly significant performance and can hardly be dismissed or considered fragmentary.

Other researchers have presented words tachistoscopically to letter-by-letter readers (Staller et al. 1978; Warrington and Shallice 1980; Patterson and Kay 1982; Prior and McCorriston 1983; Friedman and Alexander 1984). All these studies found that for letter-by-letter readers, reading comprehension requires and follows sequential letter identification; that is, they could not show the "iconic" reading process we had demonstrated in our patient. It must, however, be kept in mind that these studies, while using tachistoscopic presentation, usually presented words for a far longer time (ten times longer or more) than we did, above the threshold for conscious verbal awareness of single letters. We consider exposures below this threshold crucial for left-hemisphere inhibition not to occur. These studies, therefore, cannot be considered to disqualify our patient's initial iconic reading performance. Moreover, the results of these studies are not at variance with our findings, since our patient too was incapable of showing reading comprehension once he was aware of single letters and could read them. Recently, a number of researchers again found evidence for preserved reading capacities in pure alexia (Branch Coslett 1986; Shallice and Saffran 1986; Bub 1986). Using tests for lexical decision, semantic categorization, or contextual effects on letter identification they could show access to lexical meaning when a letter-by-letter reading strategy could not be used. Some of these results, while confirming our observations, are at variance with the report (Patterson and Kay 1982) of letter-by-letter readers' failure in lexical decision and semantic categorization.

The different and sometimes contradictory findings concerning access to lexical meaning in letter-by-letter readers may be explained not only by the differences in experimental techniques employed and theoretical positions of the experimenters, but also by the considerable individual variation among the different patients with this syndrome. In the last few years we have examined a number of patients with left posterior lesions due to various causes and with various degrees of reading disturbances. We were not able in all these patients to demonstrate access to lexical meaning when a letter-by-letter strategy was not employed, although we examined most of them tachistoscopically with a broad variety of stimuli including words and letters. A major obstacle to the demonstration of lexical meaning comprehension in our patients was the reluctance of some to guess because they were not verbally aware of having seen anything. Another difficulty was the large variation in performance between different patients at different exposure durations. If one believes that right-hemispheric access to lexical meaning is dependent on diminished control by the dominant left hemisphere, it is not unexpected to find access to lexical meaning to be dependent on exposure duration. As we have already pointed out, short exposure duration in combination with a partial anatomical disconnection may add up to a complete functional disconnection in a pure alexia.

The following case (Regard and Landis 1987; Landis 1987) may exemplify these considerations. A 62-year-old, right-handed man had a long history of adult-onset insulin-dependent diabetes mellitus and moderate alcohol intake. Three weeks prior to admission he complained of impaired vision, misreaching for objects, and a general feeling of unsteadiness and vertigo. At admission he was oriented in time and place, but somewhat slow in responding. He had an incomplete right homonymous hemianopia, reduced swing of his right arm when walking, signs of a mild polyneuropathy with reduced sensation below the knees, and no ankle jerks. Upon mental examination his speech was found to be fluent with occasional circumlocutions and word finding difficulties, but without paraphasia. Comprehension and repetition were normal. He had mild naming difficulties for the faces of famous persons, but he had no color anomia; writing was fluent, but he omitted letters and displaced words spatially. He had a complete alexia for words, but could read some single letters and numbers; he had no apraxia, agnosia or acalculia. CT scan revealed a large lesion occupying the left occipitotemporoparietal space.

This patient was treated with 12 mg of dexamethasone daily; within 3 days his writing normalized and his single letter reading improved. At this time when tested with tachistoscopic presentations, he showed classical alexia without agraphia and with an inability to read words as a whole, but with preserved letter-by-letter and auditory reading, i.e., recognition of words spelled aloud to him. Twelve days after admission the tumor, histologically a glioblastoma multiforme, was removed through a left occipital craniotomy. Three months later the patient was readmitted because he had developed a right sensorimotor hemisyndrome. Upon mental examination he showed a complete alexia with agraphia and an anomic aphasia. CT scan showed a recurrence of the tumor. Within the next 6 weeks the patient became severely aphasic with fluent paraphasic speech and impaired comprehension and repetition. At autopsy, pathology studies showed diffuse infiltration of nearly the entire left hemisphere but no infiltration of the right hemisphere.

Tachistoscopic testing was performed on the 5th and 6th day after the first admission while the patient displayed a pure alexia and a right homonymous hemianopia. His intact left visual field/right hemisphere (LVF/RH) received an array of stimuli, including single letters, concrete nouns, color patches, pictures of objects, and signs and symbols at five different exposure durations (unlimited, 500, 100, 50, and 20 ms).

As shown in Fig. 1, he read or named all stimuli except signs and symbols at unlimited exposure. To read concrete four- and five-letter nouns he used a letter-by-letter strategy. Thus his performance dropped dramatically when exposure duration was reduced. At 500 ms he read only 4 out of 12 exposed words and at 100 ms only 1 out of 12 words. He read single letters much better. At exposures as short as 20 ms he could still read 2 out of 10 single letters and, similar to the earlier described patient with pure alexia (Landis et al. 1980), this patient could not match nouns to objects when he was verbally aware of individual letters. While colors were named and matched equally poorly, pictures of objects were matched at much shorter exposure durations than they were named (complete object anomia at 50 ms, but 10 out of 12 correct picture-to-

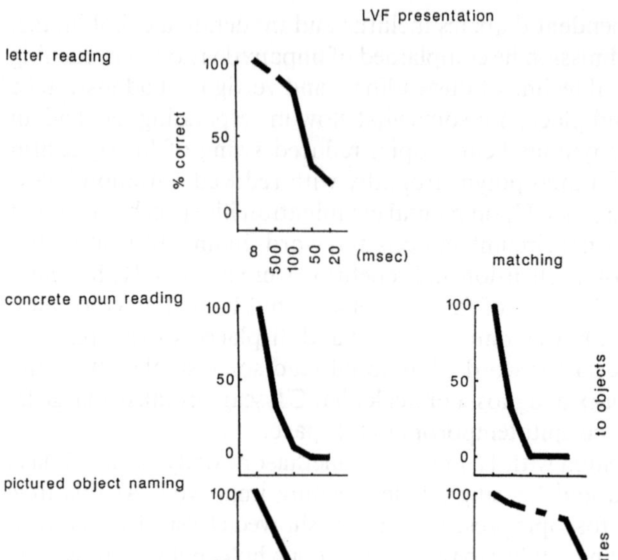

Fig. 1. Reading, naming, and matching performance (% correct) during tachistoscopic stimulus presentation to the LVF at different exposure durations (unlimited, 500, 100, 50 and 20 ms)

picture matching at 20 ms and 7 out of 12 correct at 10 ms). This latter performance shows comprehension of complex visual information in the absence of precise verbal/lexical knowledge, since at such short exposures he could neither read object names, match object names with pictures, nor name pictures of objects. When presented at reduced exposure durations with abstract and concrete German nouns of *high emotional content* [i.e., *Liebe* (love), *Hass*

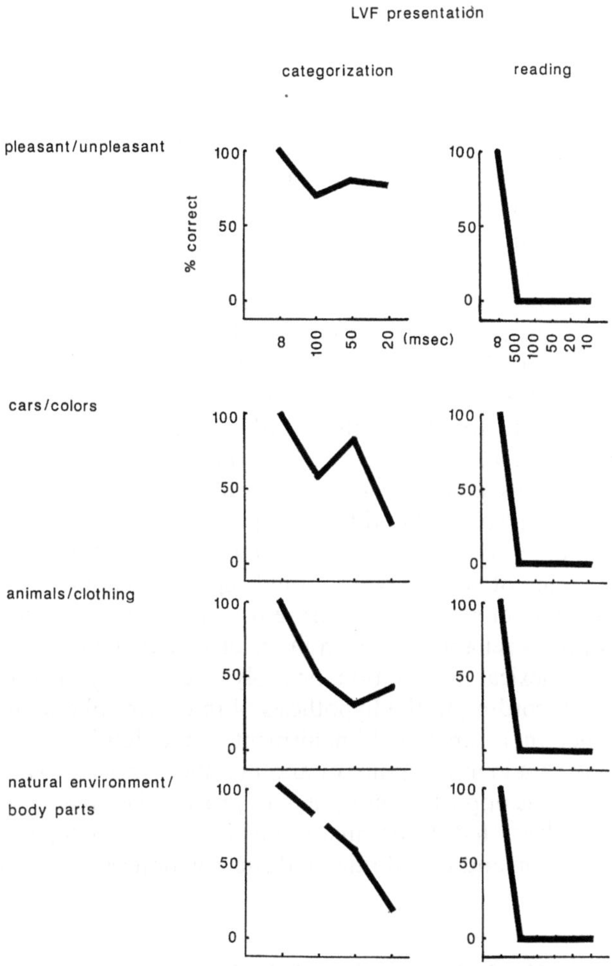

Fig. 2. Performance in word categorization and word reading (% correct) during tachistoscopic word presentation in the LVF at different exposure durations (in ms)

(hatred), *Kuss* (kiss), *Mord* (murder) etc.], however, he could not read them but spontaneously produced approving or disapproving grunts, as if he had some knowledge of the meaning of these words.

To investigate if he had *semantic* knowledge sufficient for word categorization at exposure durations where reading and even word–picture matching was impossible, we tachistoscopically presented lists of words at different exposure durations (unlimited, 100, 50, 20 ms). Each word list was made up of words from two categories and was presented in random order several times at each exposure duration. The patient was forced to choose between the two categories after each presentation even when unable to read the word or even when claiming not to have seen anything. There were four word lists each with twelve German nouns three to five letters long and with six words in each category. The categories were: (1) emotionally positive, pleasant (e.g., Love, Kiss)/emotionally negative, unpleasant (e.g., Hate, Murder); (2) cars/colors (i.e., Volvo/Green); (3) animals/clothing (i.e., Dog/Hat); (4) natural environment/body parts (i.e., Lake/Nose).

As can be seen in Fig. 2, the patient could read and categorize these words only at unlimited exposures. There was, however, one exception: his reliable *emotional* categorization of pleasant or unpleasant nouns. He correctly indicated the emotional category to which these words belonged at very short exposures (70% at 100 ms, 80% at 50 ms, 77% at 20 ms) where even single letter recognition was impaired. This demonstrates that some aspects of semantic knowledge about a written word can be maintained in the absence of correct reading aloud, single letter recognition, or verbal awareness. Again we suggest that in this patient with a clinically incomplete posterior *anatomical* disconnection syndrome the difficulty produced by decreased exposure duration amounted to a complete *functional* disconnection. Knowledge of emotional meaning of written words could represent another facet of right-hemisphere reading comprehension. Moreover, the patient's failure to categorize other concepts reliably argues in favor of specific reading comprehension for *emotional* lexical information, possibly mediated by the right hemisphere.

According to the hypothesis of interhemispheric inhibition and release of function, a functional impairment of the dominant hemisphere for a certain task should at one point or another uncover a coexisting, but inhibited capacity of the opposite hemisphere to process the same task. In the patients tested we believe that the dominant function had been impaired by a combination of the lesion and the additional difficulty induced by reduced exposure time.

Right-Hemisphere Reading: Aphasia

The notion of interhemispheric inhibition and release should hold not only for the rare pure alexic patients, but for all patients with reading disturbances due to a lesion of the language-dominant left hemisphere; that means for aphasic-alexic patients as well. Studying a group of unselected aphasic patients with left-hemisphere lesions, we could show (Landis et al. 1983) that the occurrence of semantic paralexia in these patients was dependent on lesion size and location. There are many more semantic paralexias for words presented tachistoscopically to the right hemisphere than for those presented to the left hemisphere in normal subjects (Regard and Landis 1984; Bopp 1985). Thus, we interpreted the fact that semantic paralexias occurred with larger and more posteriorly placed left-hemisphere lesions in aphasia in terms of the inhibition and release model.

Any complete disconnection of the neural substrate dominant for reading or for making lexical decisions from its homologous area in the nondominant right hemisphere should release access to lexical meaning in the latter. Therefore, any lesion destroying this dominant reading substrate completely should enable us to demonstrate right-hemispheric access to lexical meaning. In order not to test only (right-hemispheric) aspects of words such as concreteness, imageability, or emotionality we chose to use *double simultaneous* go/no-go tachistoscopic lexical decision with function words. Function words are known to be the most difficult class of words for aphasic patients to process, and we have recently shown that normal subjects perform only as well as chance allows when these function words are presented to the right hemisphere (Regard et al. 1985).

Severe reading disturbances, usually due to large lesions in the left, dominant hemispheres, are common in global aphasia. We recently assessed such a patient. This 46-year-old, right-handed man suffered a massive embolic stroke in the left middle cerebral artery during cardiac surgery, resulting in global aphasia and right sensorimotor hemisyndrome. When admitted 1 year later for treatment of focal and secondary generalized seizures about once every two months, his ambulation had improved to the point that he could walk with leg braces and a cane but his global aphasia remained. His spontaneous speech consisted largely of unintelligible dysarthric utterances. Occasionally the patient produced a contextually appropriate word, which he then perseverated. Naming, repetition, reading, and writing were extremely poor. Auditory comprehension was reduced to one-step commands. He made excellent use of pantomime, intonation, and gestures to communicate and was helped by the melody of a familiar tune to produce the corresponding words. He produced semantic paralexias and paragraphias. We tested this patient with a tachistoscopic lexical decision experiment with function words as already described.

As shown in Fig. 3 we found that this severely aphasic patient who could not read function words aloud or understand their meaning in written context could detect them as real German words in his right visual field/left hemisphere (RVF/LH) at 150 ms exposure as well as normal controls. With reduced exposure durations (50 and 20 ms) the RVF/LH performance dropped and later, in a second run at 150 ms, no learning effect could be shown. When these function words are presented to the LVF/RH, normal subjects perform this task at *chance* at exposures of 150, 100, and 50 ms (Regard et al. 1985). Our patient, however, detected function words in his LVF/RH at all exposure durations, even at 20 ms, above the 1 SD range of the performance of normal controls. More important, during the second run at 150 ms, he showed a learning effect.

These results demonstrate that under specific conditions the right hemisphere manifests some reading ability, in particular the capacity to detect function words among nonsense words. This capacity cannot be demonstrated in normal subjects with an intact left hemisphere under the same conditions, and

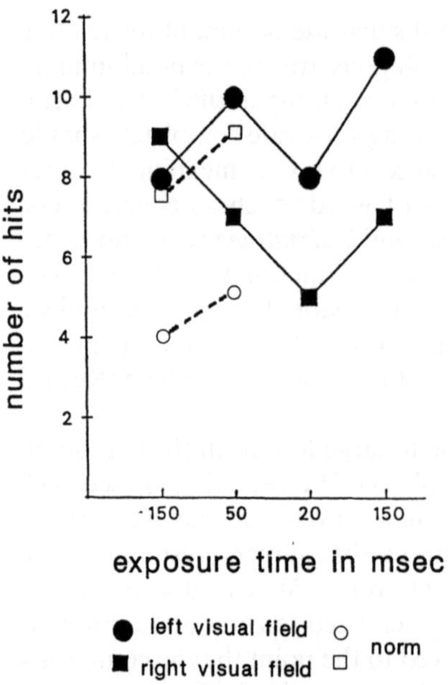

Fig. 3. Performance of a globally aphasic patient in a double simultaneous tachistoscopic lexical decision task with function words at different exposure durations: 150, 50 and 20 ms. *Solid circles* represent the left visual and *solid squares* the right visual field. *Open circles* and *squares* represent the performance of 24 normal subjects

the findings in this patient imply that the large left frontotemporoparietal infarct not only rendered this patient globally aphasic, but is responsible for the improved RH performance. Furthermore, this experiment suggests that learning of this lexical decision task occurred in the RH, but not in the LH, pointing to the activation of a neural substrate not previously used for lexical decisions.

We retested this patient recently and found at 150 ms exposure a function word detection rate of 100% in the LVF and 67% in the RVF, a performance almost identical to that obtained several months earlier, probably indicating retention of learned performance in the LVF. In the first run at 150 ms exposure both LH and RH processing seem to coexist, but subsequently a decrease in LH performance is accompanied by an increase in RH performance. Again a model of dual brain balance which postulates separate but interacting hemispheric processing systems may best explain these data.

This patient was noted to have an inferior right homonymous quadrantanopia with the smallest light marks only on Goldman perimetry. The question arose whether the impaired lexical decision performance in the RVF/LH was due primarily to a visual disturbance, not allowing enough visual information to reach the LH-processing system, or if it was due to a stimulus- or task-specific overloading of this damaged LH system. Thus, we conducted several additional experiments. (1) We presented the patient with the above lexical decision experiment again, but now only a single word or nonsense word was flashed at a time, either in the LVF or the RVF at either 150 or 50 ms. At

150 ms his performance was equally good in both visual fields (92%). At 50 ms performance remained good in the LVF (92%), but dropped to chance in the RVF. This result is compatible with both explanations. (2) We repeated the initial double simultaneous lexical decision experiment with function words, but presented the stimulus words once 2° above and once 2° below the fixation point. Therefore the right-sided stimulus was projected once in the upper quadrant of the RVF (i.e., the part of the RVF without impairment on Goldman perimetry), and once in the lower quadrant of the RVF (i.e., the part of the RVF with a field cut for the smallest light stimuli). Since we found no difference in performance between the presentation in the upper or lower RVF quadrant, a primary visual disturbance is unlikely to be the only explanation of the results. (3) We presented both at 150 and at 50 ms a lateralized test with objects of different shapes that had to be compared on the basis of their common meaning. This test has been shown to elicit a RVF/LH advantage in normal subjects (Landis et al. 1979). The patient showed a consistent RVF/LH advantage (RVF 92%, LVF 67% at 150 ms; RVF 80%, LVF 70% at 50 ms). This result suggests that it is not the primary visual disturbance, but the selective overloading of the damaged LH system which leads to the impaired RVF lexical decision performance. This in turn may lead to a release of the RH capacity for lexical decision and ultimately to learning and consolidation of this no longer "inhibited" or "controlled" ability.

Summary and Conclusions

We have tried to confirm, extend, and generalize the notion of a balance of interhemispheric inhibition and release of function with respect to reading by presenting two new experimentally investigated single cases in the framework of earlier experimental and clinical findings and some anecdotal observations. Our starting point was the observation (Landis et al. 1980) of a letter-by-letter reader, who, when prevented from using single letter information in an experimental situation, had access to lexical meaning (shown by making correct word object matches), but when able to use single letter information, had no access to the meaning of the word. We deduced that two types of reading strategies must exist; we called the first iconic reading, the second visual–verbal reading and proposed that there is no access to iconic reading as long as visual–verbal reading is available.

This observation fits the model of interhemispheric inhibition and release as initially proposed by Wigan (1844) over a century ago. In this model the hemisphere dominant for a certain function controls the opposite hemisphere's attempt to deal with the same information and prevents it from being manifested. Applied to reading, this would mean that right-hemispheric, nondominant access to lexical meaning should be demonstrated in conditions where left-hemispheric, dominant reading is abolished. This left-hemisphere function can be impaired by lesion, by experimental manipulations, or by a combination of both.

Our first new case shows that when left-hemispheric reading in a letter-by-letter reader is rendered impossible by the combination of a left posterior lesion and extremely reduced exposure duration, emotional categorization of words that cannot be read or consciously verbally understood is possible. This shows that under certain circumstances access to probably right-hemispheric lexical meaning is gained. Since it should be possible to generalize the model of interhemispheric inhibition and release, the model should also apply to all cases in which reading is impaired by a lesion of the dominant reading substrate, as is the case in alexic aphasics.

Our second detailed case demonstrates that a globally aphasic patient is, under certain experimental circumstances, able to learn to detect function words as real words in his nondominant left visual field, but fails to do so in his dominant right visual field. This second case, together with our data from normal subjects (Regard et al. 1984, 1985), we believe, permits application of the interhemispheric inhibition and release of function model to explain different reading strategies, and suggests that this may be a general model to explain dual brain interaction.

Acknowledgements. We thank Dr. Dorothea Weniger for her help in testing the aphasic patient, Dr. Jane Casey for her critical comments and editorial help, and Elisabeth Häsler for typing the manuscript.

References

Assal G, Regli (1980) Syndrome de disconnexion visuo-verbale et visuo-gestuelle. Rev Neurol (Paris) 136:365–376

Benson DF (1985) Alexia. In: Vinken PJ, Bruyn GM, Klawans HL (eds) Handbook of clinical neurology, vol 1 (45). North-Holland, Amsterdam, pp 433–455

Benson DF, Geschwind N (1969) The alexias. In: Vinken PJ, Bruyn GM (eds) Handbook of clinical neurology, vol 4. North-Holland, Amsterdam, pp 112–140

Bopp B (1985) Lesestrategie der rechten und linken Hemisphäre. Diplomarbeit, Psychologie, University of Freiburg im Breisgau

Branch Coslett H (1986) Preservation of lexical access in alexia without agraphia. J Clin Exp Neuropsychol 8(2):146

Bub D (1986) Access to the word-form system in letter-by-letter readers. J Clin Exp Neuropsychol 8(2):146

Campbell R, Landis T, Regard M (1986) Face recognition and lipreading. A neurological dissociation. Brain 109:509–521

Caplan LR, Hedley-Whyte T (1974) Cuing and memory dysfunction in alexia without agraphia. Brain 97:251–262

Damasio AR, Damasio H (1983) The anatomical basis of pure alexia and color "agnosia". Neurology 33:1573–1583

Day J (1977) Right-hemisphere language processing in normal right handers. J Exp Psychol [Hum Percept] 3:518–528

Dejerine J (1892) Contribution a l'etude anatomo-pathologique et clinique des differentes varietes de cecite verbale. CR Seances Mem Soc Biol 44:61–90

Dixon NF (1981) Preconscious processing. Wiley, London
Ellis HD, Shepherd JW (1974) Recognition of abstract and concrete words presented in the left and right visual fields. J Exp Psychol 103:1035–1036
Friedman RB, Alexander MP (1984) Pictures, images and pure alexia: a case study. Cogn Neuropsychol 1:9–23
Geschwind N (1965) Disconnexion syndromes in animals and man (part I). Brain 88:237–294
Graves R, Landis T, Goodglass H (1981) Laterality and sex differences for visual recognition of emotional and non-emotional words. Neuropsychologia 19:95–102
Greenblatt SH (1977) Neurosurgery and the anatomy of reading: a practical review. Neurosurgery 1:6–15
Holender D (1986) Semantic activation without conscious identification in dichotic listening, parafoveal vision, and visual masking: a survey and appraisal. Behav Brain Sci 9:1–66
Kreindler A, Ionasescu V (1961) A case of "pure" word blindness. J Neurol Neurosurg Psychiatry 24:275–280
Landis T (1987) Right hemisphere reading: A clinico-experimental approach to the dual brain interaction. Habilitationsschrift, University of Zürich
Landis T, Assal G, Perret E (1979) Opposite cerebral hemispheric superiorities for visual associative processing of emotional facial expressions and objects. Nature 278:739–740
Landis T, Regard M (in press) Two cases of prosopagnosia and alexia. Part I. In: Bajic M (ed) Advances in the Bio science. Pergamon, Oxford
Landis T, Regard M, Serrat A (1980) Iconic reading in a case of alexia without agraphia by a brain tumor: a tachistoscopic study. Brain Lang 11:45–53
Landis T, Regard M, Graves R, Goodglass H (1983) Semantic paralexia: a release of right hemispheric function from left hemispheric control. Neuropsychologia 21:359–364
Moscovitch M (1976) On the representation of language in the right hemisphere of right-handed people. Brain Lang 3:47–71
Patterson K, Besner D (1984a) Is the right hemisphere literate? Cogn Neuropsychol 1:315–341
Patterson K, Besner D (1984b) Reading from the left: a reply to Rabinowics and Moscovitch and to Zaidel and Schweiger. Cogn Neuropsychol 1:365–380
Patterson K, Kay J (1982) Letter-by-letter reading: psychological descriptions of a neurological syndrome. Q J Exp Psychol [A] 34:411–441
Prior M, McCorriston M (1983) Acquired and developmental spelling dystexia. Brain Lang 20:263–285
Regard M, Landis T (1984) Experimentally induced semantic paralexias in normals: a property of the right hemisphere. Cortex 20:263–270
Regard M, Landis T (1987) Emotional word categorization in a pure alexic patient. J Clin Exp Neuropsychol 9:40–41
Regard M, Landis T, Graves R (1985a) Dissociated hemispheric superiorities for reading stenography vs print. Neuropsychologia 23:431–435
Regard M, Landis T, Wieser HG, Hailemariam S (1985b) Functional inhibition and release: unilateral tachistoscopic performance and stereoencephalographic activity in a case with left limbic status epilepticus. Neuropsychologia 23:575–581
Regard M, Stodieck SRG, Landis T, Wieser HG (1986) Temporary shift from left to right hemisphere dominance in lexical decisions caused by seizure. J Clin Exp Neuropsychol 8(2):127
Richardson JTE (1975) The effect of word imageability in acquired dyslexia. Neuropsychologia 13:281–287
Shallice T, Saffran E (1986) Lexical processing in the absence of explicit word identification: evidence from a letter-by-letter reader. Cogn Neuropsychol 3:439–458
Smith A (1966) Speech and other functions after left (dominant) hemispherectomy. J Neurol Neurosurg Psychiatry 29:467–471

Sperry RW, Gazzaniga MS, Bogen JE (1969) Interhemispheric relationships: the neocortical commissures; syndromes of hemispheric disconnection. In: Vinken PJ, Bruyn GW (eds) Handbook of clinical neurology, vol 4. North-Holland. Amsterdam, pp 273–290
Stachowiak FJ, Poeck K (1976) Functional disconnection in pure alexia and color naming deficit demonstrated by deblocking methods. Brain Lang 3:135–143
Staller J, Buchanan D, Singer M, Lappin J, Webb W (1978) Alexia without agraphia: an experimental case study. Brain Lang 5:378–387
Warrington EK, Shallice T (1980) Word-form dyslexia. Brain 103:99–122
Wigan AL (1844) Duality of the mind. Longman, Brown, Green and Longman, London (Simon reprint, 1985)
Zaidel E (1978) Lexical organization in the right hemisphere. In: Buser PA, Rougeul Buser A (eds) Cerebral correlates of conscious experience. INSERM symposium no 6. Elsevier/North-Holland, Amsterdam, pp 177–197
Zaidel E (1985) Right hemisphere language. In: Benson DF, Zaidel E (eds) The dual brain. Guilford, New York

The Variability of Right-Hemisphere Reading Capacities in Global Aphasia *

DOROTHEA WENIGER, VIVIAN KITTERINGHAM and MIRJAM EGLIN

Introduction

The reading performance of patients with the acquired reading disorder known as deep dyslexia has given rise to much discussion in recent years. The issue of concern is whether the residual reading skills of these patients reflect functioning islands of the impaired left hemisphere or (normally available) processing mechanisms of the intact right hemisphere (cf. Patterson and Besner 1984; Zaidel and Schweiger 1984). Proponents of the latter view assume that the right hemisphere possesses some ability to access lexical information from print and that this ability becomes operative when the preferred processing mechanisms of the left hemisphere cease to be available. Since the right hemisphere has been found incapable of deriving phonology from print (Moscovitch 1976; Zaidel and Peters 1981) the reading competence of the right hemisphere is limited. Whenever a phonological code has to be assembled from orthographic input (as, for example, in reading nonsense words or in making rhyme judgments) the solution of the task appears to depend on left-hemisphere structures.

Although there can be little doubt that the right hemisphere is capable of lexical-semantic processing, the evidence from visual half-field studies with normal individuals remains inconclusive as to the characteristics of vocabulary items to which the right hemisphere is sensitive with a certain degree of constancy across individuals. As Patterson and Besner (1984) point out in their brief review of the visual laterality studies in which concreteness/imageability effects were examined, strong biases towards concrete words are not found consistently in the left visual field (LVF)/right hemisphere (RH). Methodological differences between the studies could be responsible for this lack of consistency, but it is just as likely that the inconsistent experimental findings reflect individual differences in the organization of the RH lexicon. Since the RH lexicon appears to be more experientially structured and far less amenable to logical and linguistic concepts than the LH lexicon (Marcel and Patterson 1978; Zaidel 1978), such differences defy controlled study.

One of the main points of criticism which Patterson and Besner (1984) have raised against the adoption of a RH reading system is that "no predictable

* This study was supported by the Swiss Science Foundation, grant numbers 3.852-0.85 and 3.828-0.86.

level of skill and pattern of characteristics" (p. 336) has been demonstrated in patients supposedly displaying RH reading. In their reply to such criticism Zaidel and Schweiger (1984, 1985) argue that the variable participation of the RH, which is observed in the reading performance of deep dyslexics, presumably reflects a breakdown in the mechanisms regulating the assignment of reading control. The authors base their arguments on the view that normal reading calls for a controlled coordination of interhemispheric interaction and that in brain-damaged individuals this coordination becomes disrupted. However, brain lesions commonly result in rather variable disruptions of cognitive functions so that a regulation model is probably too general to account for psychological data with any interesting degree of predictability.

The evidence reported in support of a RH reading hypothesis is usually based on studies with brain-damaged individuals. It is of course a truism that *no* hypothesis about the residual reading skills of a damaged brain can be generalized to the reading performance of a normal brain. It would seem, though, that more insight could be gained from available sources if attention were directed toward those psychological parameters which could be responsible for the variations in RH reading. Particularly in global aphasic patients one would expect to find signs of RH reading – at least on the basis of a regulation model as proposed by Zaidel and Schweiger (1984). If such expectations turn out to be unwarranted, we might want to examine whether the absence of the expected skills could have something to do with the extent and pattern of the patients' language impairments. Such an approach could provide some data on how impaired language functions affect reading performance. It is, however, not without methodological drawbacks. Global aphasic patients usually have large LH lesions so that any LVF advantage obtained in a linguistic task could be a matter of LH degradation rather than RH dominance. Adequate control tasks are required to ascertain that perceptual deficits cannot (fully) account for the visual field advantages. The aim of this study is to examine the RH reading abilities of global aphasic patients in a word recognition task under conditions of unilateral and bilateral stimulation and to relate the established skills to the extent and pattern of language impairment.

Word Recognition with Unilateral Stimulation

Our study is based on the assumption that the ability of global aphasic patients to recognize and understand written words involves RH processing mechanisms – to some variable degree. The assumption is supported by a number of studies on language recovery which suggest a relationship between degree of impairment and RH involvement. For example, in some dichotic listening studies with aphasic subjects a left ear advantage was found for verbal stimuli (Johnson et al. 1977; Pettit and Noll 1979; Castro-Caldas and Botelho 1980); this inversion of the ear advantage tends to be encountered in aphasics with severe language deficits. Using the Wada Test, Czopf (1972) has also found that severely impaired aphasics displayed an almost complete disruption of their residual language abilities after the injection of sodium amytal into the right carotid artery; less severely impaired aphasics only showed a mild disruption of their recovered language skills. Although most of these patients have extensive lesions in the language area of the LH, size of lesion is probably not the decisive variable (cf. Niccum et al. 1983).

In our attempts to determine which of the two hemispheres is better in recognizing written words we used the technique of lateralized stimulus presentation. The method allows one to assess differences in the processing of stimuli presented to the left and right visual field (LVF and RVF). But, as Moscovitch (1986) discusses in his review of visual laterality studies, these differences can be interpreted along quite different lines, depending on the model of laterality adopted (e.g., from notions of interhemispheric transfer to concepts of differential hemispheric arousal). In patients with unilateral brain damage the interpretation of such differences becomes even more intricate because lesion-related changes in attentional capacity or resource allocation could have produced them. This is a crucial point in split-field studies, to which we shall return. It is important to note that control tests utilized to ascertain that no gross perceptual deficits in either visual field are affecting performance do not contribute to an understanding of such issues of reorganization.

The stimulus material consisted of 36 words, 2 from each of 18 semantic categories. One of the two words from a semantic category represented a prototypical member, the other a nonprototypical one (Weniger and Schmid 1979). The decision to use prototypicality as a stimulus variable was motivated by the lack of sufficiently large lists of nouns rated for concreteness, familiarity, or meaningfulness in German. The length of the stimulus words varied from four to six letters. They were all printed in capitals (Helvetica 18 Point). The point nearest the center of the viewing screen was 1.7° of visual angle from the center. A black dot in the center of a blank field was used as the fixation point, visible except when a word was projected to a visual field. A headrest ensured a constant viewing distance of 48 cm. The multiple choice set of pictures in which the meaning of the presented words had to be identified consisted of six line drawings. One line drawing depicted the stimulus word, the remaining five depicted objects from the same semantic category as the target and represented either prototypic or nonprototypic members with respect to the stimulus word.

Subjects were instructed on each trial to look directly at the fixation point and keep their eyes fixed on it until after a word had been presented to either the LVF or the RVF. After stimulus presentation they were to select the meaning of the presented word from the multiple choice set placed to the right of the apparatus. Each of the 36 words was presented twice in randomized order, once to each visual field, at an exposure of 150 ms. Stimulus words never appeared more than three consecutive times in the same visual field. To familiarize subjects with the procedure they were given a set of practice trials.

Table 1. Sample characteristics of subjects

	Age (years)	Duration (months)	Diagnostic test scores[a]				
			Token test	Repetition	Written language	Naming	Comprehension
E.v.H.	46	21	5	16	18	16	11
H. J.	51	14	10	18	19	0	37
W. Z.	61	12	16	13	20	6	30
A. L.	48	38	16	27	20	6	21
H. D.	58	18	19	35	5	42	26
G. Z.	51	51	28	58	51	41	61
H. F.	65	40	36	49	20	42	30
E. P.	58	60	39	11	31	15	56
E. M.	53	52	42	33	34	42	31

[a] Percentile rank scores (Aachen Aphasia Test).

Nine global aphasic patients with no gross perceptual deficits in either visual field participated in the study. Sample characteristics are given in Table 1. In this table patients are listed in the order of their percentile rank scores on the Token Test (standardized German version with correction for age; Orgass 1976).

At first glance one might suspect a certain relationship between degree of severity as measured by the Token Test and onset of aphasia. But since the patients with an aphasia of longer duration have been achieving almost the same test scores over an extended period of time, it is rather unreasonable to correlate degree of recovery with duration of illness. A comparison of the patients' diagnostic test scores does reveal some points to consider when evaluating their performance in the word recognition task. Patient E.P. achieved almost the best level of performance on the Token Test and in (auditory and written) comprehension tasks, but had poorer scores than most of the other patients in tasks calling for an oral response (repetition, confrontation naming, oral reading). The linguistic deficits characterizing this patient's aphasia appear to be tied up with pronounced motor-speech problems. This probably also holds for H.J., whose Token Test score is much lower than E.P.'s. In contrast to E.P., the patient H.D. did rather well in tasks with oral responses but achieved the lowest score in the subtest "written language." This subtest of the Aachen Aphasia Test comprises three groups of tasks, namely, reading words and sentences aloud, assembling letters and words to words and sentences, and writing dictated words and sentences (cf. Willmes et al. 1983).

The percentage of correct identifications are given in Figs. 1 and 2, separately for each subject. No significant visual field effects were found either for the prototypical (Fig. 1) or the nonprototypical (Fig. 2) words. The more severely impaired subjects tend to identify prototypical words in the LVF correctly more often, whereas in the less impaired subjects better performances

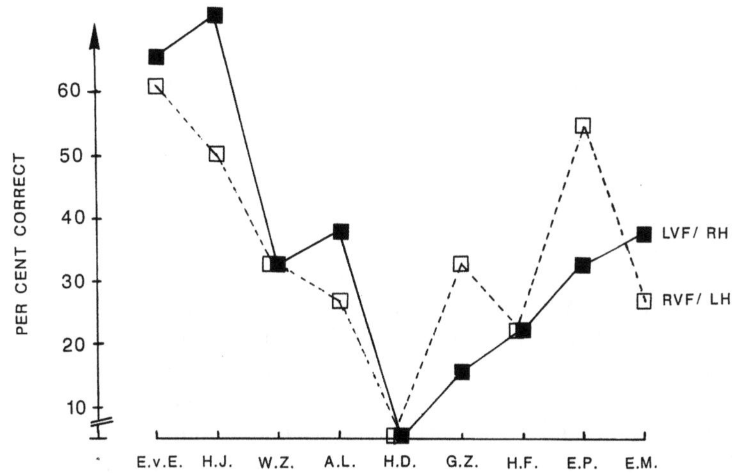

Fig. 1. Identification of prototypical words with unilateral stimulation at 150 ms

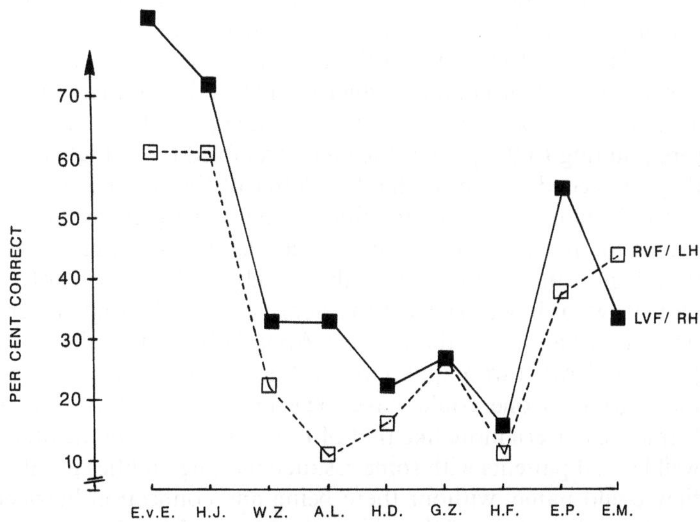

Fig. 2. Identification of nonprototypical words with unilateral stimulation at 150 ms

are observed for the prototypical words in the RVF. With nonprototypical words most patients do better when the stimulus words are presented in the LVF. Some numerical differences might favor the LVF: although the medians for the number of correct identifications are just about the same in the four experimental conditions, the upper range of performance lies higher with words presented to the LVF. The highest level of performance was achieved by the two patients with the lowest Token Test scores.

A RVF advantage is generally obtained in word recognition studies with normal subjects, the degree of asymmetry being a matter of stimulus conditions and presentation mode (unilateral versus bilateral; cf. Beaumont 1982). As has been suggested (Hines 1975), the variability of the asymmetries found may be the result of selective channeling: with some types of words the two hemispheres operate as independent processing channels, with other types transmission to the LH takes place. This line of reasoning leaves us with two possible interpretations. It could be that words were processed in the hemisphere to which they were projected. The decreased level of performance observed in the RVF reflects the lesion effect. But it might also be that for words in the RVF there was a transfer of information from the left hemisphere to the intact right hemisphere. Such a transfer appears to have been most effective in the two patients with the lowest Token Test scores, at least judging from the fact that their level of performance is higher than that of the other patients. This observation seems to support the assumption that RH reading involves a release of LH control (cf. Zaidel and Schweiger 1985; Landis and Regard, this volume).

One could argue that patients W.Z., A.L., H.D., G.Z., and H.F. tended to perform below or around chance level because reading control was maintained in the damaged LH. Three of these five patients (H.D., G.Z., H.F.) attempted to solve the task in a manner which could be taken as indirect evidence for such a claim. These patients often tried to name all pictures in the array aloud before pointing to the picture they felt resembled the stimulus word. Sometimes they succeeded in naming the first letter of the stimulus word and then used this information as a cue for finding the target picture. This strategy can be successful in "recovering" the "missed" letters of a stimulus word – provided that there is an intact naming ability to rely on. It is worth noting that the three patients who showed signs of this achieved considerably higher scores on confrontation naming in the Aachen Aphasia Test than the other two patients (W.Z. and A.L.) who apparently did not adopt such a response strategy. On these grounds one could have expected W.Z. and A.L. to display a performance pattern more like that of E.v.E. and H.J. On the other hand it might well be that patients with some residual naming abilities pointed to the picture they could name, without there being any connection between the stimulus word and the name of the object they pointed to. Such a response behavior is tantamount to selecting the most appealing picture. The strikingly poor performance of H.D. in identifying prototypical stimulus words could reflect this. Supportive evidence is given by the following observation: When a group of normal subjects ($n=8$) was asked to point to the picture in each array which appealed most, the target picture was selected on the average of 8.3% – just about the level of H.D.'s performance.

The findings of our word recognition task provide no conclusive evidence as to whether independent hemispheric processing or information transfer is taking place in the individual aphasic subjects of the study. The observed response strategies suggest that the extent to which particular linguistic functions are impaired can have its effects on how a given linguistic task is executed (cf. Moscovitch 1986). It is surely reasonable to assume that the impaired language system adapts itself differentially, depending on task demands and cognitive resources. Instead of viewing hemispheric differences in terms of control assignment to one of the two hemispheres, it could be more enlightening to examine them in terms of response strategies.

Word Recognition with Bilateral Stimulation

Bilateral stimulation has been found to enhance the visual field advantages obtained under conditions of unilateral stimulation (Rosen et al. 1975). If the two hemispheres operate as independent channels, no such enhancement is to be expected. If interhemispheric transfer is necessary, there will be information loss in transfer and in delay, resulting in an increased visual field advantage for stimuli processed in the hemisphere of input. To find out whether the aphasic patients were relying on processing mechanisms of the RH to the same extent, they were given a word recognition task under conditions of bilateral stimulus presentation.

The stimulus material consisted of 36 pairs of words. These were compiled from a set of words comprised of two prototypical and two nonprototypical members from each of the 18 semantic categories used in the first experiment. Both words of a pair were either prototypical or nonprototypical and did not have any obvious semantic relationship to each other (e.g. *Löwe*, lion, and *Arzt*, doctor; *Kohl*, cabbage, and *Bahn*, train). They were matched for length as well as possible. With most word pairs (75%) the two words were the same length; with pairs of unequal length the difference was never more than one letter. The words in two-thirds of the pairs were either four or five letters in length; in the remaining third they were five or six letters long. Typeface was the same as in the first experiment and the point nearest the center of the viewing screen was again 1,7° of visual angle from the center. The multiple choice set of line drawings comprised a depiction of each of the two stimulus words and four distractors, two for each stimulus word. The distractors were depictions of objects from the same semantic category as the particular stimulus word and represented either prototypical or nonprototypical members according to the stimulus word.

The procedure was basically the same as in the task with unilateral stimulation. The word pairs were presented twice in such a way that each word of a pair appeared once in the LVF and once in the RVF. The order in which the meaning of the two words had to be identified was not controlled (and in our subjects could not be controlled). As can be seen in Figs. 3 and 4 the expected effects of bilateral stimulation were found.

All patients (with a single exception) correctly identified more words presented to the LVF. The three patients with the lowest Token Test scores and

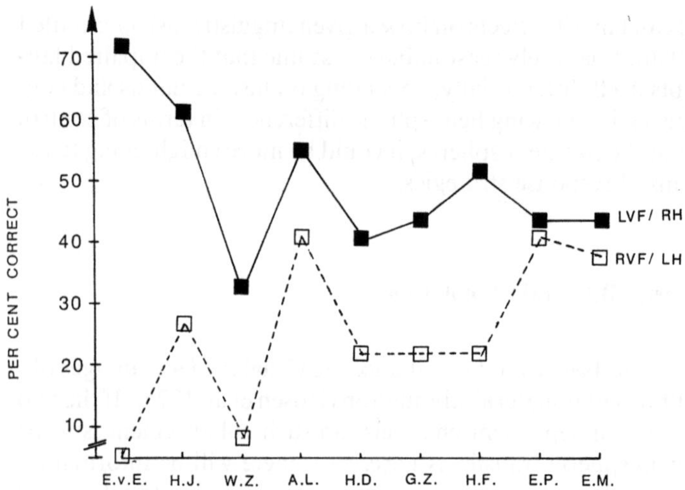

Fig. 3. Identification of prototypical words with bilateral stimulation at 150 ms

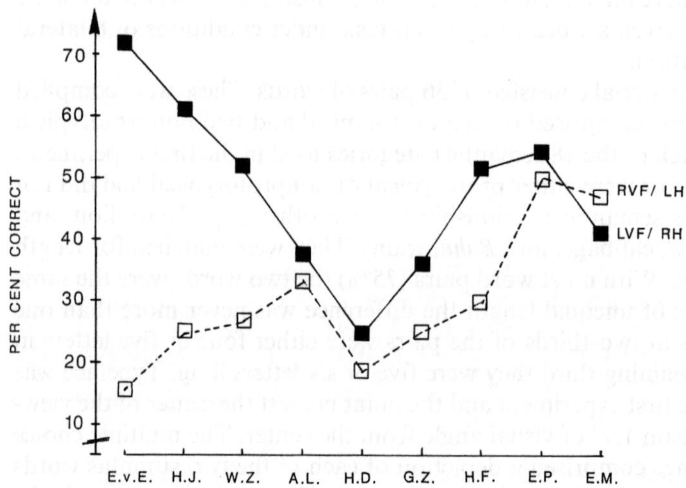

Fig. 4. Identification of nonprototypical words with bilateral stimulation at 150 ms

the poorest overall performance on a diagnostic aphasia test showed a significant LVF advantage for the two types of stimulus words ($P < 0.05$; McNemar Test with continuity correction). In three further patients (H.D., G.Z., and H.F.) the LVF superiority reached or just missed the level of significance only with prototypical words.

The results of the bilateral condition seem to point to RH involvement in word recognition. In the unilateral condition almost the same mean level of performance was observed in the two visual fields; in the bilateral condition a considerably larger mean number of correct identifications was found for words presented in the LVF than for words presented in the RVF. On the one hand, these findings may be regarded as supportive evidence for more efficient processing of words presented in the LVF. On the other hand, they suggest that in the unilateral condition the two hemispheres did not operate independently and that some interhemispheric transfer must have occurred. However, one can only speculate on what might have been going on. The data certainly do not reflect an overall triggering of RH reading as may be inferred from the range in the level of LVF performance. With unilateral stimulation no significant correlation was found between the severity of language impairment and the magnitude of the visual field difference in the number of correct identifications. As only one word was presented at a time in the unilateral condition there was no competition for the use of the available processing resources. Words in one visual field might still have had privileged access because these resources are concentrated in one hemisphere, making interhemispheric transfer necessary. Under conditions of bilateral stimulation the correlation between the degree of language impairment and the magnitude of the visual field differences proved significant for both prototypical and nonprototypical words ($r_s = 0.75$ and $r_s = 0.73$, respectively; $P < 0.05$).

Perhaps a more adequate approach to an understanding of the experimental findings is to discuss them in terms of notions developed in resource theory. Resource theory describes performance on a given task as a function of subject-task parameters imposed on the information processing system and the processing facilities controlled by this system (cf. Navon and Gopher 1979). Subject-task parameters comprise task characteristics such as stimulus type, exposure duration, visual field of presentation, response mode, etc. Depending on task characteristics particular processing resources are demanded. Given the adaptiveness of the brain as an information processing system, subjects are assumed to have at their disposal a variety of alternative means to achieve successful performance. It is therefore possible for subjects using resource compositions which are quite distinct from each other to attain similar levels of performance. In Friedman and Polson's (1981) account of resource theory the two hemispheres are conceived as separate processing systems with a fixed and limited resource supply that is inaccessible to the other hemisphere. The attempt is made to examine laterality effects with regards to differences in resource allocation. Many tasks can probably be performed successfully by both hemispheres, each hemisphere making use primarily of its own processing mechanisms and resources. The processes or mechanisms used by the two hemispheres may be the same or similar, but in order to achieve equal levels of performance in a particular task, different amounts of resources might be required. There may also be tasks for which different processes or mechanisms are used in the two hemispheres. If the resources applied to them are equal in amount and efficiency, both hemispheres could perform similarly. As the authors conjecture, such a single-task situation seems tenable in a number of studies in which letters, words, shapes, or faces had to be matched on the basis of their physical identity.

What do these considerations infer with regard to the performance of the aphasic subjects in the two word recognition tasks? The recognition and identification of words is generally associated with an RVF advantage, but depending on the linguistic characteristics of the verbal stimuli, the RH has been found to display comparable processing abilities. Familiar concrete nouns demonstrate this in particular (Day 1977). It is therefore reasonable to assume that the tasks in our study can be performed by both hemispheres of the normal brain. Let us further assume that each hemisphere performs the tasks by using some combination of its own mechanisms and resources, but that the hemispheric resource compositions are differentially efficacious. The lesion in aphasic subjects reduces the resources available in the LH. The residual resource capacity will allow only deficient processing. The issue of concern, however, is whether the processing which the LH is still capable of doing draws on supplies of the RH. With simultaneous stimulation of the two visual fields significant LVF advantages were obtained in the more severely impaired aphasic subjects; in addition, the visual field differences were larger in patients with a greater overall degree of impairment. This could mean that as LH resources become more limited (as a consequence of brain damage), supplies of the RH are drawn on more heavily. If the RH is engaged in performing the same task as the LH, a capacity limit is reached. The number of correct responses given to words presented in the RVF under conditions of bilateral stimulation therefore decreases with increasing demands for RH supplies. Under conditions of unilateral stimulation RH supplies can be drawn on with less constraint, resulting in smaller visual field differences in patients with lower diagnostic test scores.

Credible as this discussion of our findings in terms of notions from resource theory may seem, it nevertheless raises questions concerning the scientific merit of the theory. Unless it allows us to make reasonably precise predictions about behavioral phenomena, it provides us with little more than useful metaphors (for a critical review of resource theory see Navon 1984). Unilateral brain damage may be assumed to have an effect on the perceptual asymmetries obtained in studies with normal subjects. This effect is inevitably tied up with a lesion-related reduction in resource capacity. Depending on the cortical structures affected by the lesion there will be limitations on the processes or mechanisms available and the changes in perceptual asymmetries will vary accordingly. The extent to which such variations can be adequately captured within the conceptual framework of resource theory has yet to be examined.

Conclusion

As expected, LVF advantages were generally obtained in the two word recognition experiments. However, these reached a significant level only under conditions of bilateral stimulation. Reliable signs of RH reading were found in the more severely impaired aphasic subjects. As the correlation between performance level and overall degree of language impairment suggests, the RH contribution in reading processes are more likely to be observed among the severe global aphasics. But since there was considerable variation among the individual aphasic subjects in the number of words correctly identified in the two visual fields, both with unilateral and bilateral stimulation, such quantitative approaches in the interpretation of LVF advantages need to be supplemented by qualitative ones. The reported experiments did not control for the possibility that subjects might be directing their attention differently to the two visual fields. In a pilot study with the patient H.J. we obtained a shift in visual field advantages by means of instructional attention manipulation. As Hardyck et al. (1985) demonstrated in a series of lexical decision tasks, subject-directed shifts in attention do not lead to changes in visual field asymmetry. Whether this is valid to the same extent in brain-damaged subjects needs yet to be examined. It might well be that brain-damaged subjects seek to by-pass their processing difficulties by focusing their attention on formal aspects of the experimental procedure or on the stimulus materials which happen to "catch their eye" in order to produce some response. It was suggested that notions of resource theory are best suited to account for the variation in the magnitude of the obtained LVF advantages. This should be accompanied by careful control of response behavior.

There is likely to have been individual variation in the premorbid hemispheric organization of language in the brain-damaged subjects studied. As has been shown by Chiarello et al. (1984) group lateralization effects are frequently not reflected in the responses of the individual subjects to the laterally presented stimuli. A complex set of factors appears to contribute to the variability of RH reading. A regulation model probably explains only part of the story.

References

Beaumont JG (1982) Studies with verbal stimuli: In: Beaumont JG (ed) Divided visual field studies of cerebral organization. Academic, New York

Castro-Caldas A, Botelho MAS (1980) Dichotic listening in the recovery of aphasia after stroke. Brain Lang 10:145–151

Chiarello C, Dronkers N, Hardyck C (1984) Choosing sides: on the variability of language lateralization in normal subjects. Neuropsychologia 22:363–373

Czopf J (1972) Über die Rolle der nichtdominanten Hemisphäre in der Restitution der Sprache der Aphasischen. Arch Psychiatr Nervenkr 216:162–171

Day J (1977) Right-hemisphere language processing in normal right-handers. J Exp Psychol [Hum Percept] 3:518–528

Friedman A, Polson M (1981) Hemispheres as independent resource systems: limited-capacity processing and cerebral specialization. J Exp Psychol [Hum Percept] 5:1031–1058

Hardyck C, Chiarello C, Dronkers NF, Simpson GV (1985) Orienting attention within visual fields: how efficient is interhemispheric transfer? J Exp Psychol [Hum Percept] 11:650–666

Hines D (1975) Independent functioning of the two cerebral hemispheres for recognizing bilaterally presented tachistoscopic visual half-field stimuli. Cortex 11:132–143
Johnson JP, Sommers RK, Weidner WE (1977) Dichotic ear preference in aphasia. J Speech Hear Res 20:116–129
Marcel AJ, Patterson K (1978) Word recognition and production: reciprocity in clinical and normal studies. In: Requin J (ed) Attention and performance, vol VII. Erlbaum, Hillsdale, NJ
Moscovitch M (1976) On the representation of language in the right hemisphere of right-handed people. Brain Lang 3:47–71
Moscovitch M (1986) Afferent and efferent models of visual perceptual asymmetries: theoretical and empirical implications. Neuropsychologia 24:91–114
Navon D (1984) Resources – a theoretical soup stone. Psychol Rev 91:216–234
Navon D, Gopher D (1979) On the economy of the human processing system. Psychol Rev 86:214–255
Niccum N, Rubens AB, Selnes OA (1983) Dichotic listening performance, language impairment, and lesion location in aphasic listeners. J Speech Hear Res 26:42–49
Orgass B (1976) Eine Revision des Token Tests, Teil I und II. Diagnostica 22:70–87, 141–156
Patterson K, Besner D (1984) Is the right hemisphere literate. Cogn Neuropsychol 1:315–341
Pettit JM, Noll JD (1979) Cerebral dominance in aphasia recovery. Brain Lang 7:191–200
Rosen JJ, Curcio F, MacKavey W, Herbert J (1975) Superior recall of letters in the right visual field with bilateral presentation and partial report. Cortex 11:144–154
Weniger D, Schmid M (1979) Einfluß der Prototypikalität auf die Verfügbarkeit von Wörtern bei Aphasie. Project report to the Deutsche Forschungsgemeinschaft
Willmes K, Poeck K, Weniger D, Huber W (1983) Facet theory applied to the construction and validation of the Aachen Aphasia Test. Brain Lang 18:259–276
Zaidel E (1978) Lexical organization in the right hemisphere. In: Buser P, Rougeul-Buser A (eds) Cerebral correlates of conscious experience. Elsevier/North Holland, Amsterdam
Zaidel E, Peters AM (1981) Phonological encoding and ideographic reading by the disconnected right hemisphere: two case studies. Brain Lang 14:205–234
Zaidel E, Schweiger A (1984) On wrong hypothesis about the right hemisphere: commentary on K. Patterson and D. Besner, "Is the right hemisphere literate?". Cogn Neuropsychol 1:351–364
Zaidel E, Schweiger A (1985) Right hemisphere reading: a case of "déjà lu". Behav Brain Sci 8:365–367

Semantic Priming in the Intact Brain: Separate Roles for the Right and Left Hemispheres? *

CHRISTINE CHIARELLO

Introduction

In this chapter evidence is considered about lateralized lexical processing in the intact brain obtained when the visual pathways leading to one cerebral hemisphere are selectively stimulated [the visual half-field (VHF) method – see Beaumont 1982]. Such studies have yielded considerable information about hemisphere differences in word recognition processes (see Chiarello, in press, for review). In the realm of semantics, most investigations have attempted to delineate the *kinds of words* (i.e., concrete, emotional) that the right hemisphere can recognize. The research I describe here takes a different tack. Our focus is on the *processes available* to each hemisphere for accessing word meanings and semantic relationships between words. Accessing knowledge about semantic relatedness, the linking of word meanings via association or semantic similarity, is an important aspect of language comprehension. If the hemispheres differ in how lexical-semantic relations are processed, this would also have consequences for "higher order" semantic operations which depend on the availability of this lexical knowledge.

This work addresses two broad questions in an attempt to reconcile left-hemisphere (LH) language predominance with the growing list of right-hemisphere (RH) language abilities. (1) What specific processes are available to the left hemisphere alone to enable it to predominate in overall language function despite an apparent hemispheric equality in some linguistic domains? It may be that only a few linguistic functions are strictly lateralized to the left hemisphere, but that these are crucial for adequate language performance. (2) What language processes are available to the right hemisphere, and under what circumstances might these be utilized despite the presence of similar information in the left hemisphere? The data to be discussed here suggest that while both hemispheres contribute to lexical-semantic processing, some processes are strictly lateralized to the left hemisphere (i.e., semantic inhibition), while others are bihemispheric (semantic facilitation). Further, we describe conditions under which certain lexical information may be more accessible to the right hemisphere than to the left.

This chapter begins by describing the theoretical rationale for the semantic priming techniques which we have employed and then presents the results of

* This research was supported by BSRG Grant S07 RR077068-19.

this research. Next, these findings are compared to other relevant VHF research and a unifying hypothesis is proposed to account for the hemisphere differences in lexical-semantic processing which are found when studying the normal brain. Finally, speculations are made on the separate roles of the right and left hemispheres during normal language processing and suggestions about how the proposed hypothesis would account for some of the semantic deficits seen after RH brain injury are offerred.

Semantic Priming

In our laboratory we have been using semantic priming techniques to investigate the locus of hemisphere differences in lexical-semantic processing. When a word to be recognized is preceded by a semantically related word, its processing is facilitated (in speed and accuracy) relative to conditions where the preceding item is not semantically related (Neely 1976; Fischler 1977). Two mechanisms, each acting under different conditions, can account for such semantic priming: spreading activation and controlled semantic processing (Neely 1977; Seidenberg et al. 1984). Our interest is in how these two mechanisms are utilized by the left and right hemispheres.

To understand the spreading activation process, it is necessary to consider how information is organized in semantic memory. Semantic memory can be viewed as a network structure with semantically related concepts directly linked within the network (Collins and Loftus 1975). Recognition of a word will activate a corresponding representation in the network, and some of this activation will spread, via links in the network, to representations of semantically related words. If one of these related items is then presented, its recognition is facilitated. Thus, this spreading activation process temporarily produces a set of related concepts having an increased activation level. For a time, these activated items will be more available for subsequent processing. However, processing of unrelated words will be unaffected since their activation levels will not have changed.

Spreading activation priming can be considered a relatively automatic process in that the effect occurs regardless of the subject's expectancies about prime–target relatedness (Neely 1977; Humphreys 1985). It is characterized by facilitation *without* inhibition for unrelated words and can be demonstrated when the prime is pattern-masked (Marcel and Patterson 1978; Fowler et al. 1981), when there is a very brief interval between prime and target words (Fischler and Goodman 1978), or when the proportion of related primes is small (Fischler 1977).

The second kind of priming, controlled priming, occurs whenever the subject actively processes the meaning of the prime to develop semantic expectancies about possible target words (Tweedy et al. 1977). When an expected (related) word appears, its processing is facilitated since attention has been directed to a relevant area of semantic memory (Neely 1976, 1977). However, when an unexpected (unrelated) word is shown, processing is inhibited. That is, subjects are slower to respond than in a neutral, baseline condition due to the violation of expectancies and the misdirection of attention. Controlled priming can be demonstrated when there is a prime–target interval of 400 ms or greater (Neely 1977) or when there is a high probability of semantically related prime–target pairs in the experiment (Tweedy et al. 1977).

Our research indicates that the semantic processes underlying these two kinds of priming are not equally available to each hemisphere (Chiarello 1985; Chiarello et al. 1987). In these studies we altered subjects' semantic expectancies by varying the proportion of trials in which semantically related primes appeared. With a low proportion (25%) of related primes it is difficult for subjects to actively use the prime as a semantic predictor of the target since most prime–target pairs are completely unrelated. Thus, subjects are unlikely to develop an expectancy about possible target words and should not use the prime to focus attention on a set of semantically related terms. Priming obtained under these conditions should reflect an automatic spreading activation process. We can contrast these effects with those obtained using a high proportion (75%) of related primes. To encourage an expectancy about likely target words, we instructed subjects to focus attention on the meaning of the prime word, treating it as a high probability predictor of possible target words. Priming obtained under these conditions should reflect a more attention-demanding, controlled semantic process, with facilitation for related words *and* inhibition for unrelated words.

In addition to related and unrelated word primes, neutral primes (XXXX or BLANK) were included to serve as a baseline condition. Such primes are considered neutral because they have no semantic associates. By comparing related and unrelated trials to the neutral condition, we can determine whether priming is due to facilitation (related trials faster than neutral) or inhibition (unrelated trials slower than neutral). While facilitation is expected for both high and low probability priming, inhibition should only occur under controlled, high probability prime conditions.

In these experiments, right-handed college students were randomly assigned to either low or high probability prime conditions. The target was tachistoscopically presented in either the RVF or LVF, 500 ms after presentation of the prime word. Subjects made lexical decisions about the target strings, which were either familiar words or pronounceable nonwords. Reaction time (RT), measured from onset of the target, is the dependent variable of interest.

In an initial study (Chiarello 1985), related stimulus paris were members of the same semantic category (INCH–YARD). Table 1 shows the overall priming effect (RT unrelated – RT related) we observed in each VF/H. Similar effects were obtained for accuracy. As always, words were recognized faster, and more accurately, in the RVF. Yet, as shown here, priming was not invariably larger in the RVF. These data suggest that the direction of hemisphere

Table 1. Semantic priming for high and low probability conditions by VF (Chiarello 1985)

	Low probability		High probability	
	LVF	RVF	LVF	RVF
Priming (ms)	+61	+17	+60	+85

Table 2. Facilitation, inhibition, and overall priming (ms) by VF (Chiarello et al. 1987)

	Low probability		High probability	
	LVF	RVF	LVF	RVF
Facilitation	+23	+21	+61	+ 40
Inhibition	(− 6)	(− 4)	(−14)	− 61
Priming	+29	+25	+75	+101

Nonsignificant effects are given in parentheses.

differences in priming depends on whether or not subjects can adopt a semantic expectancy.

The neutral prime employed in this study (XXXX) proved to be unsuitable in that the longest RTs occurred in this condition (see also deGroot et al. 1982; Patton and Lefton 1985). Thus, we could not differentiate facilitation from inhibition processes in this study. However, low probability semantic priming was larger in the LVF, and high probability priming larger in the RVF. This may indicate a more potent spread of activation in the RH, although the LH appears better able to use expectancies to focus attention on a cohort of semantically related words.

We undertook a second study (Chiarello et al. 1987) which incorporated some methodological improvements. A lexical neutral prime (BLANK) was used in place of XXXX, and related targets were semantic associates of their primes (POLICE–JAIL). The results of this study are shown in Table 2. Because the BLANK neutral prime did not yield excessively long RTs, this condition could be used to separate facilitation from inhibition priming. Facilitation is calculated by (RT neutral – RT related), inhibition by (RT neutral – RT unrelated), and overall priming by (RT unrelated – RT related). Thus, facilitation occurs whenever related trials are *faster* than neutral, while inhibition is present whenever unrelated trials are *slower* than neutral.

As Table 2 indicates, under low probability conditions priming was due entirely to facilitation, as would be expected for an automatic spreading activation process. Further, there is no hemispheric asymmetry for this effect as most other investigations of VF automatic semantic priming have reported (Marcel

Table 3. Laterality effects in the size of semantic priming obtained in VHF studies permitting separation of automatic and controlled processes

	Automatic	Controlled
Marcel and Patterson 1978	=VF	—
Chiarello 1985	>LVF	>RVF
Walker and Ceci 1985, Exp. 2	=VF	—
Chiarello et al. 1987	=VF	>RVF
Burgess and Simpson 1988a	=VF	>RVF
Eglin 1987	=VF	—

Dashes indicate that controlled priming was not assessed.

and Patterson 1978; Walker and Ceci 1985; Eglin 1987). Thus, the previous finding of greater LVF low probability priming was not replicated. We are currently investigating whether this discrepancy is due to the differing semantic relations used in the two studies. For now it is important to note that in neither study was automatic, low probability priming greater in the RVF/LH.

For high probability priming, greater priming was obtained in the RVF as in our previous study. Note that RVF priming was a function of both inhibition and facilitation, as predicted for an expectancy-based, controlled priming effect. However, there was no inhibition for unrelated trials in the LVF (the 14 ms apparent inhibition did not even approach significance, $F < 1$). Thus it appears that at least one aspect of controlled semantic processing, inhibition for unexpected, unrelated words, may be specific to the LH. These results suggest that semantic spreading activation occurs in both hemispheres, but that only the left hemisphere makes use of expectancies to process semantics in a focal manner, facilitating the processing of some items and actively inhibiting others.

Our findings are consistent with those obtained in other lateralization studies of semantic priming. Table 3 summarizes the results of those VHF studies in which automatic and controlled priming effects could be distinguished.[1] Although these investigations involved different subjects, stimuli, and different ways of assessing automatic versus controlled priming, the results are remark-

[1] There are some additional VHF priming experiments (Zaidel 1983; Walker and Ceci 1985, Exp. 1) which were not designed to separate the effects of spreading activation from more controlled semantic processing. Since we cannot ascertain whether the results are attributable to automatic or controlled priming processes, these studies are not considered here. Zaidel (1983, this volume) has reported inhibitory semantic priming in the LVF. However, the neutral condition Zaidel employed may not be appropriate for assessing true semantic inhibition: no primes occurred in the baseline condition which was measured in a separate test session with a separate group of subjects. Since viewing any two stimuli in close temporal proximity may slow recognition of the second item, comparing unrelated prime trials to an "unprimed" baseline may result in a spurious inhibition effect, for reasons having little to do with *semantic* processing.

ably similar. It is evident that controlled priming, characterized by semantic inhibition for unrelated words, is consistently greater in the RVF. It is equally evident that automatic priming, which is believed to be due to the spreading activation process, is never greater in the RVF.

The results of Burgess and Simpson (1988 a) are especially interesting. In their study ambiguous words were used as primes, and they varied the interval between the prime and target. Most studies show that, while all meanings of an ambiguous word are available at a point relatively early in the process, eventually only the dominant or contextually appropriate sense remains available (Swinney 1979; Seidenberg et al. 1982). Burgess and Simpson showed that this latter process occurred only in the LH, via active inhibition of the subordinate meaning. At the longest prime–target interval (750 ms) there was significant facilitation for both dominant and subordinate meanings in the RH, while in the LH only the dominant meaning was facilitated with inhibition of the subordinate meaning (i.e., performance below that for unrelated trials). In other words, at a time when the left hemisphere had selected one appropriate meaning and supressed all others, the right hemisphere was still maintaining multiple interpretations.

Lateralization of Semantic Processing: A Hypothesis

The VHF semantic priming results lead to an intriguing hypothesis about hemisphere differences in the processing of semantic relations. The data suggest that right hemisphere semantics may be characterized by a lack of selectivity, while the left hemisphere semantic system is more finely tuned, focusing on a particular interpretation and inhibiting all others. Thus, the RH maintains several activated meanings, while the LH has focused on only one. This is consistent with our findings that only the LH is capable of controlled semantic processing, although initial semantic activation of a network of relations occurs in both hemispheres. Since there is little evidence for semantic inhibition in the RH, this initial activation of multiple meanings and semantic relations could well persist for some time in the RH. This suggests that the RH may play a role in maintaining "background" semantic information which is not immediately relevant.

Some converging evidence comes from visual half-field studies of Stroop interference. If RH semantic processing operates without selection, then Stroop-like interference should be restricted to the LH, since it results from the necessity to *select* one response from others which are simultaneously activated (Dyer 1973). The typical Stroop color–word interference effect for English orthography is significantly larger in the RVF/LH (Schmit and Davis 1974; Tsao et al. 1979; Hugdahl and Franzon 1985), implying that activation of an irrelevant color word interferes with selection of the appropriate color name primarily in the LH. Lupker and Sanders (1982) demonstrated that picture–word interference in the RVF/LH was potentiated when the distractor word was semantically related to the picture, whereas in the LVF/RH interference due to a semantically related word was no greater than that observed for any letter string. This suggests that interference based on competing semantic information only occurs in the left hemisphere (see also Zaidel, this volume). The Stroop data are consistent with the hypothesis that the LH functions to select from among several candidate semantic representations the one which will receive further processing.

Thus, I am proposing that semantic processing in the LH operates in a *focal* manner with enhanced processing of relevant meanings, but suppression (inhibition) of meanings which, although related, are not currently relevant. In contrast, the RH processes semantic relations in a *nonfocal* manner with rather widespread facilitation of related meanings, but without selectivity. That is, within the set of meanings activated in the RH, none receives preferential processing at the expense of the others.

This distinction is reminiscent of the focal–diffuse dichotomy which Semmes (1968) proposed some years ago to account for hemisphere differences in the representation of elementary sensory and motor functions (see also Gur et al. 1980). However, there is an important difference between these two proposals. We make no claim that lexical information is *represented* (i.e., localized) more focally in the left hemisphere than the right, or that the RH employs a more diffuse (i.e., distributed) means of representing the same information. Our argument rests solely on hemisphere differences in the pattern of activation and inhibition which exists among related word meanings, independent of whether the meanings themselves are represented in a focal or distributed fashion (the representation issue is discussed by Rumelhart and McClelland 1986). We propose that by using inhibition as well as facilitation the LH *processes* meaning focally, while the RH, having no access to such inhibitory processes, cannot focus on a single interpretation in preference to other related meanings.

It is also important to point out that our hypothesis concerns the facilitation and inhibition of semantic information *within each hemisphere*, and as such is quite different from proposals that right-hemisphere language processing is normally inhibited by the dominant LH (i.e., *interhemispheric* inhibition, see Landis and Regard, and Zaidel, this volume). Undoubtedly, interhemispheric cooperation is necessary to coordinate access to the differing patterns of *intrahemispheric* semantic activation which we posit (see also Burgess and Simpson, 1988b). The specifics of this hemispheric coordination remain to be worked out [2], but it is argued here that RH semantic activation does play a role in normal language comprehension.

What might be the function of this rather diffuse RH semantic system for normal language processing? We might expect the RH to arrive at a general

[2] It is of some interest that one theory of interhemispheric function, the "topographic inhibition" model (Cook 1986), has independently postulated RH and LH semantic networks having properties similar to those described here (see Cook 1986, Chap. 4).

conception of meaning but to be unable to focus on the most appropriate interpretation from a set of likely candidates. Thus, exclusive use of the RH semantic system would result in a preponderance of semantic errors or paralexias, a possibility which has already received considerable attention (e.g., Coltheart 1980; Landis et al. 1983; Marshall and Patterson 1983). Yet certainly the RH, in and of itself, could not support normal language comprehension, which would require a much higher degree of semantic specificity.

However, we should also consider the consequences of total reliance on the LH system. Since it appears that nonfocal meanings or concepts are actively suppressed or inhibited in the left hemisphere, any situation requiring semantic reanalysis or simultaneous consideration of more than one level of meaning would be problematic. Examples of such situations would be reinterpreting "garden path" sentences, understanding jokes or double entendres, indirect speech acts, etc. However, if alternate meanings were still activated in the RH, one could quickly recover additional interpretations simply by accessing the RH system.

This view provides a conceptual framework for interpreting some of the semantic deficits which have been reported for RH-lesioned patients. Although such individuals have no across-the-board comprehension deficits, they are impaired in interpreting more subtle aspects of linguistic meaning (Wapner et al. 1981). For example, RH-injured patients have difficulty in appreciating connotative aspects of meaning (Brownell et al. 1984), jokes (Brownell et al. 1983; Bihrle et al. 1986), indirect speech acts (Foldi 1987), ambiguity (Brownell, this volume), and metaphor (Winner and Gardner 1977). It has recently been shown that such patients find it particularly difficult to revise an initial interpretation in light of subsequent, contradictory information (Brownell et al. 1986). Thus, they tend to get "locked in" to a single interpretation of a word, sentence, or discourse. I suggest that this is diagnostic of overreliance on LH semantics, as articulated here. After RH injury there would be no backup system to access when an initial interpretation must be revised. This would manifest itself as an inability to reevaluate meaning, since in the only remaining semantic system, that of the left hemisphere, active suppression of nonfocal meanings would be occurring. Although undoubtedly other deficits contribute to the difficulties RH-lesioned patients have in semantic processing, the hypothesis proposed here suggests a mechanism which may underlie many aspects of the RH language syndrome.

Conclusions

To summarize, I have presented evidence that automatic semantic activation takes place in either hemisphere, but that some aspects of controlled semantic processing depend on a normally functioning left hemisphere. These results, in conjunction with other related research, suggest that the LH utilizes semantic inhibition as well as semantic facilitation to yield a single, relevant interpretation. Since the RH appears to lack this inhibitory mechanism, multiple interpretations which were initially activated could persist in parallel with the left hemisphere's one select meaning. In the normal brain, this RH semantic system can be accessed whenever it is necessary to revise or supplement an earlier interpretation. However, because RH semantics is diffuse and nonselective, it could not support normal semantic processing after profound LH injury. By the same token, semantic processing would not be entirely normal after RH injury either. Due to overreliance on the left hemisphere's more focal, selective semantics, we would expect deficits whenever an initial interpretation had to be revised or supplemented.

This interpretation is clearly quite speculative, but it is consistent with a great deal of evidence about lateralization of semantic processing in the normal brain and the consequences of unilateral brain injury. Additional study will be required to further test and refine these ideas. Regardless of the ultimate interpretation, there can be little doubt that the coordinated functioning of both cerebral hemispheres is necessary to support the full range of lexical semantic processing.

Acknowledgments. I am grateful to Lorie Gage and Alma Pollock for their comments on this manuscript.

References

Beaumont JG (ed) (1982) Divided visual field studies of cerebral organization. Academic, London

Bihrle AM, Brownell HH, Powelson JA, Gardner H (1986) Comprehension of humorous and nonhumorous materials by left and right brain-damaged patients. Brain Cogn 5:399–411

Brownell HH, Michel D, Powelson J, Gardner H (1983). Surprise but not coherence: sensitivity to verbal humor in right-hemisphere patients. Brain Lang 18:20–27

Brownell HH, Potter HH, Michelow D, Gardner H (1984) Sensitivity to lexical denotation and connotation in brain-damaged patients: a double dissociation? Brain Lang 22:253–265

Brownell HH, Potter HH, Bihrle AM, Gardner H (1986) Inference deficits in right brain-damaged patients. Brain Lang 27:310–321

Burgess C, Simpson GB (1988 a). Cerebral hemispheric mechanisms in the retrieval of ambiguous word meanings. Brain Lang 33:86–103

Burgess C, Simpson GB (1988 b). Neuropsychology of lexical ambiguity resolution: the contribution of divided visual field studies. In: Small SL, Cottrell GW, Tanenhaus MK (eds) Lexical ambiguity resolution in the comprehension of human language. Morgan Kaufmann, Los Altos

Chiarello C (1985) Hemisphere dynamics in lexical access: automatic and controlled priming. Brain Lang 26:146–172

Chiarello C (in press) Lateralization of lexical processes in the normal brain: a review of visual half-field research. In: Whitaker HA (ed) Contemporary reviews in neuropsychology. Springer, Berlin Heidelberg New York

Chiarello C, Senehi J, Nuding S (1987) Semantic priming with abstract and concrete words: differential asymmetry may be postlexical. Brain Lang 31:43–60

Collins AM, Loftus EF (1975) A spreading-activation theory of semantic processing. Psychol Rev 82:407–428
Coltheart M (1980) Deep dyslexia: a right-hemisphere hypothesis. In: Coltheart M, Patterson K, Marshall JC (eds) Deep dyslexia. Routledge and Kegan Paul, London, pp 326–380
Cook ND (1986) The brain code: mechanisms of information transfer and the role of the corpus callosum. Methuen, London
de Groot AMB, Thomassen JWM, Hudson PTW (1982) Associative facilitation of word recognition as measured from a neutral prime. Mem Cogn 10:358–370
Dyer FH (1973) The Stroop phenomenon and its use in the study of perceptual, cognitive, and response processes. Mem Cogn 1:106–120
Eglin M (1987) Interference and priming within and across visual fields in a lexical decision task. Neuropsychologia 25:613–624
Fischler I (1977) Associative facilitation without expectancy in a lexical decision task. J Exp Psychol [Hum Percept] 3:18–26
Fischler I, Goodman GO (1978) Latency of associative activation in memory. J Exp Psychol [Hum Percept] 4:455–470
Foldi NS (1987) Appreciation of pragmatic interpretations of indirect commands: comparison of right and left hemisphere brain-damaged patients. Brain Lang 31:88–108
Fowler CA, Wolford G, Slade R, Tassinary L (1981) Lexical access with and without awareness. J Exp Psychol [Gen] 110:341–362
Gur RC, Packer IK, Hungerbuhler JP, Reivich M, Obrist WD, Amarnek WS, Sackeim HA (1980) Differences in the distribution of gray and white matter in human cerebral hemispheres. Science 207:1226–1228
Hugdahl K, Franzon M (1985) The incongruent color-words paradigm and language lateralization: an EEG-study. Scand J Psychol 26:321–326
Humphreys GW (1985) Attention, automaticity, and autonomy in visual word processing. In Besner D, Waller TG, Mackinnon GE (eds) Reading research: advances in theory and practice, vol 5. Academic, Orlando, pp 253–310
Landis T, Regard M, Graves R, Goodglass H (1983) Semantic paralexia: a release of right hemisphere function from left hemisphere control? Neuropsychologia 21:359–364
Lupker SJ, Sanders M (1982) Visual field differences in picture-word interference. Brain Cogn 1:381–398
Marcel AJ, Patterson KE (1978) Word recognition and production: reciprocity in clinical and normal studies. In: Requin J (ed) Attention and performance, vol VII. Halsted, New York, pp 209–226
Marshall JC, Patterson KE (1983) Semantic paralexia and the wrong hemisphere: a note on Landis, Regard, Graves, and Goodglass (1983). Neuropsychologia 21:425–427
Neely JH (1976) Semantic priming and retrieval from lexical memory: evidence for facilitatory and inhibitory processes. Mem Cogn 4:648–654
Neely JH (1977) Semantic priming and retrieval from lexical memory: roles of inhibitionless spreading activation and limited-capacity attention. J Exp Psychol [Gen] 106:226–254
Patton BL, Lefton LA (1985) Facilitation without inhibition. Bull Psychon Soc 23:191–194
Rumelhart DE, McClelland JL (1986) Parallel distributed processing, vol 1. Foundations. MIT, Cambridge
Schmit V, Davis R (1974) The role of hemispheric specialization in the analysis of Stroop stimuli. Acta Psychol (Amst) 38:149–158
Seidenberg MS; Tanenhaus MK, Leiman JM, Bienkowski M (1982) Automatic access of the meanings of ambiguous words in context: some limitations of knowledge-based processing. Cogn Psychol 14:489–537
Seidenberg MS, Waters GS, Sanders M, Langer P (1984) Pre- and postlexical loci of contextual effects on word recognition. Mem Cogn 12:315–328
Semmes J (1968) Hemispheric specialization: a possible clue to mechanism. Neuropsychologia 6:11–26
Swinney D (1979) Lexical access during sentence comprehension: (re)consideration of context effects. J Verb Learn Verb Behav 14:645–660

Tsao Y, Feustelk T, Soseos C (1979) Stroop interference in the left and right visual fields. Brain Lang 8:367–371
Tweedy JR, Lapinski RH, Schvaneveldt RW (1977) Semantic context effects on word recognition: influence of varying the proportion of items presented in an appropriate context. Mem Cogn 5:84–89
Walker E, Ceci SJ (1985) Semantic priming effects for stimuli presented to the right and left visual fields. Brain Lang 25:144–159
Wapner W, Hamby S, Gardner H (1981) The role of the right hemisphere in the apprehension of complex linguistic materials. Brain Lang 14:15–33
Winner E, Gardner H (1977) The comprehension of metaphor in brain-damaged patients. Brain 100:717–729
Zaidel E (1983) Disconnection syndrome as a model for laterality effects in the normal brain. In: Hellige J (ed) Cerebral hemisphere asymmetry: method, theory and application. Praeger, New York, pp 95–151

Hemispheric Locus of Lexical Congruity Effects: Neuropsychological Reinterpretation of Psycholinguistic Results *

Eran Zaidel, Hedy White, Eriko Sakurai and William Banks

Introduction

This paper addresses two separate questions. The first is substantive and concerns the nature of normal right-hemisphere involvement in lexical semantics. Three psycholinguistic paradigms have been adapted to lateralized tachistoscopic presentation and yield new evidence on hemispheric differences and independence in automatic, i.e., involuntary and unattended, lexical processes. This illustrates the usefulness of psycholinguistics to neuropsychology.

The second question addressed in this paper is methodological. It concerns the possible advantages of structural over functional models of cognitive processes. Does localization add to our psychological understanding of a cognitive or linguistic process? Many cognitive psychologists believe that the structure of the brain is irrelevant to our understanding of the mind, much as the hardware of a particular digital computer is irrelevant to the functional flow chart of the program implemented on it. Some cognitive psychologists consider data from clinical neurological patients relevant to models of normal function, but only as sources of behavioral evidence, not as sources of useful structural information. Only few cognitive psychologists seek to articulate general principles of brain functioning in the hope that they will clarify general principles of functioning of the mind. This paper belongs in the latter category. At the very least, neuropsychological considerations constrain the class of possible functional models (Zaidel 1986). In this paper we will demonstrate that neuropsychological analysis can reinterpret classical psycholinguistic effects and show some of these effects to be incidental or structural epiphenomena. This illustrates the usefulness of neuropsychology to psycholinguistics.

Hemispheric Independence

The two cerebral hemispheres may be conceptualized as two fairly complete and independent information processing systems. Each hemisphere often represents the same input information differently and applies different strategies to it. On this view the two normal cerebral hemispheres work in parallel with

* This work was supported by NIH Grant NS-20187, by NIMH RSDA MH-00179 and by a UCLA BRSG to the first author.

occasionally conflicting results, much like in the disconnection syndromes. In order to effect unified behavior. conflicts need to be resolved and priority established by a suprahemispheric control mechanism. Much control is probably mediated by callosal facilitation and inhibition (Zaidel 1986).

There is now substantial evidence that both normal hemispheres have considerable lexical-semantic competence capable of processing both spoken and printed words (Zaidel 1985). But the organization of the lexicon in the right hemisphere (RH) is different than that of the left hemisphere (LH). In particular, the RH reading lexicon seems more diffuse, with poor demarcation between semantically related words, better representation of concrete nouns than abstract function words, and no grapheme-phoneme conversion.

The question then arises whether classical psycholinguistic semantic congruity or faciliation/inhibition effects in reading apply to either hemisphere or whether they reflect interhemispheric interaction. By "semantic congruity effects" we are referring to general symbolic match/mismatch conditions such as occur in priming experiments, Stroop-like effects, and comparative judgment tasks. If a congruity effect is shown to hold differently in each hemisphere, then does one hemisphere dominate in central presentation using the standard psycholinguistic paradigm? If a congruity effect reflects interhemispheric interaction, does it require a reinterpretation? We will illustrate the range of possible answers using three examples. The first involves a semantic-orthographic, bilingual, Stroop-like paradigm, the second involves semantic facilitation in lexical decision, and the third involves a symbolic comparative judgment task. The first example shows that different Stroop-like effects occur in each hemisphere. The second example suggests that the primary locus of semantic priming and inhibition can be unilateral, in the RH! The third example shows that congruity effects in comparative judgment require hemispheric cooperation and are often artifacts of interhemispheric transfer of sensorimotor information. A brief methodological preliminary is presented next.

Models of Laterality Effects in the Normal Brain

A right visual half-field advantage (RVFA) in a lateralized tachistoscopic experiment with linguistic stimuli may reflect, at the limit case, the effects of callosal transfer due to exclusive LH specialization (callosal relay) or, alternatively, the difference in relative processing efficiency between the two hemispheres, each processing the stimuli presented to it (direct access). One way to tell whether an observed laterality effect in normal subjects reflects callosal relay or direct access is to pair stimuli in each field with responses by either hand. Then, under certain simplifying assumptions, a significant response hand × visual field interaction would signal direct access, whether or not superimposed on a main effect showing a visual field advantage (Fig. 1). In direct access, when central processing requires all available resources and interferes with response programming in a given hemisphere, we may observe a contra-

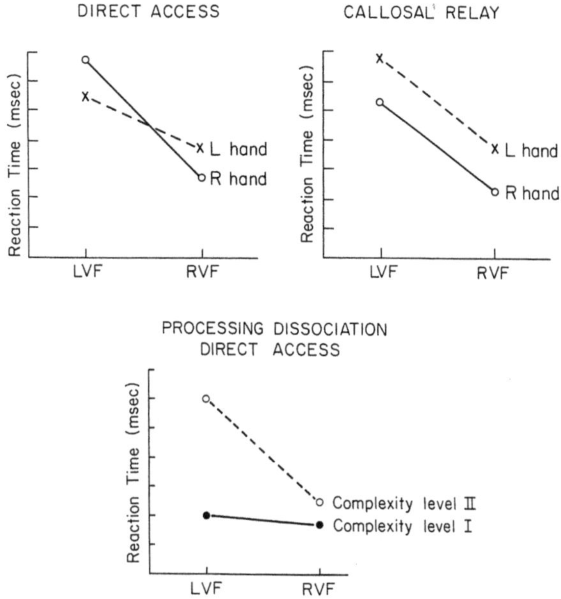

Fig. 1. Some patterns of behavioral laterality effects, in experiments with stimuli and responses restricted to one hemisphere, that are diagnostic of exclusive hemispheric specialization for the task versus independent hemispheric processing

lateral rather than ipsilateral advantage in the hand × field interaction [right hand faster in the left visual half-field (LVF) and left hand faster in the right visual half-field (RVF)]. Conversely, a significant main effect yielding a visual field advantage together with a corresponding main effect showing an ipsilateral response hand advantage (i.e., a RVFA and faster responses by the right hand or a LVFA and faster responses by the left hand) would signal callosal relay and exclusive specialization by the hemisphere opposite the superior field and hand (Zaidel 1983a; Fig. 1).

Under the usual simplifying assumptions, it can be shown theoretically that when a task combines a sequence of direct access and callosal relay components, the net hand × field pattern is callosal relay, with the VFA determined by the first callosal relay component, and the hand advantage determined by the last callosal relay component. This predicts, for example, that any naming task should show a main effect of response hand with a right hand advantage, since only the left hemisphere is believed to control speech in a normal right-handed subject. Thus, a direct access pattern reflects a process that is carried to completion in one hemisphere, i.e., all of whose components are direct access (Zaidel 1986).

Another sign of direct access is a "processing dissociation" showing a significant interaction between visual field of presentation and some binary stimulus dimension, such as concrete versus abstract nouns (Fig. 1). Unless there are different speeds of callosal transfer for the different poles of the dimension, this pattern indicates that each hemisphere applies its own characteristic information processing strategy to the same stimuli (but see Eviatar and Zaidel, 1988).

Three Examples

A Lateralized Orthographic-Semantic Bilingual Stroop-like Effect with Manual Responses

In a study done by Sakurai and Zaidel (1988) coordinate bilingual Japanese-American high school students whose native language was Japanese received lateralized English or Japanese words which meant either "English" or "Japanese." Three English and three Japanese print types were used (Fig. 2). The first English print type was a standard upper case helvetica medium 24, the second was lower case, and the third was a fancy script. The first Japanese type was the ideographic Kanji, the second was the simpler, phonotactic Hiragana, which is acquired earlier and used more commonly, and the third was the more complex, phonotactic Katakana, which is used mostly to transliterate foreign words. The task required either language identity, i.e. print, decisions ("Is the word *printed* in English or in Japanese?") or meaning decisions ("Does the word *mean* English or Japanese?") and called for a manual, binary choice between English and Japanese. On a given trial the task was signalled by an arrow at fixation, with an upward arrow indicating print decisions and a downward arrow indicating meaning decisions. Field of presentation (L,R), orthography (English upper case, English lower case, English script, Kanji, Hiragana, Katakana), meaning (English, Japanese), and task (print, decisions, meaning decisions) were changed pseudorandomly. Response hands (L,R), were changed in blocks within subjects. The experiment was conducted by Ms.

ENGLISH	JAPANESE
English	Japanese
ENGLISH	JAPANESE
英語	日本語
えいご	にほんご
エイゴ	ニホンゴ

Fig. 2. The stimuli used by Sakurai and Zaidel. One of the twelve words is flashed randomly to the left or right of fixation and the subject is required to indicate manually whether the word is printed in Japanese or in English (language identity print decisions), or whether the word means "Japanese" or "English" (meaning decisions)

Eriko Sakurai, a UCLA psychology graduate student and a native Japanese, as an independent research project.

In either language identity (print) or meaning decisions, when the print and meaning correspond to the same language (congruous condition), decisions are facilitated, whereas when the print is in one language and the word denotes the other (incongruous condition), decisions are inhibited. The latency or accuracy difference between the two conditions can be defined as the "Stroop effect." The experimental paradigm does not permit identification of the information processing stage of the Stroop effect, but the effect probably involves perceptual analysis as well as conceptual encoding and response selection (Stirling 1979). In any case, print decisions involve perceptual identification, and the Stroop effect then reflects inhibition due to automatic access of the meaning of the stimulus word, whereas meaning decisions involve lexical-semantic access, and the Stroop effect then reflects inhibition due to perceptual interference via automatic access to the response codes. Therefore, the "net Stroop effect," i.e., the Stroop effect in the print task (meaning interference) minus the Stroop effect in the meaning task (perceptual interference), may be regarded as a measure of the relative speed of automatic lexical-semantic access, corrected by perceptual identification; i.e., the net effect is a measure of semantic access relative to perceptual recognition and identification. In interpreting the net Stroop effects we may assume that if a process A (say lexical-semantic access) interferes with a process B (say perceptual identification) more than B interferes with A, then A is faster, more efficient, or more dominant than B. Thus, hemispheric differences in the net Stroop effect for a given stimulus category reflect hemispheric differences in the relative efficiency of perceptual and semantic processes for that category.

The results showed an overall hand × visual field interaction with an ipsilateral advantage (left hand faster and more accurate in the LVF, etc.) signalling a direct access task (Fig. 3). There was an overall Stroop effect showing faster responses when the print and meaning match (e.g., the word "Japanese" printed in Japanese) and slower responses when the print and meaning are in conflict (e.g., the word "English" printed in Japanese; Fig. 4). There was also a similar and significant Stroop effect for each task and each visual hemifield.

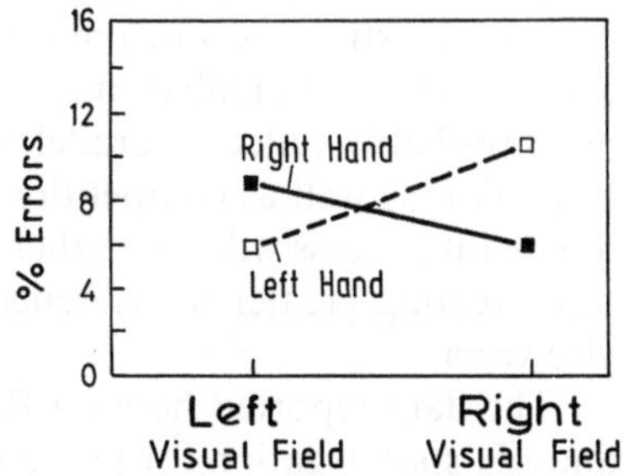

Fig. 3. Response hand by visual field interaction of overall error scores in the bilingual Stroop experiment, signaling direct access or independent hemispheric processing

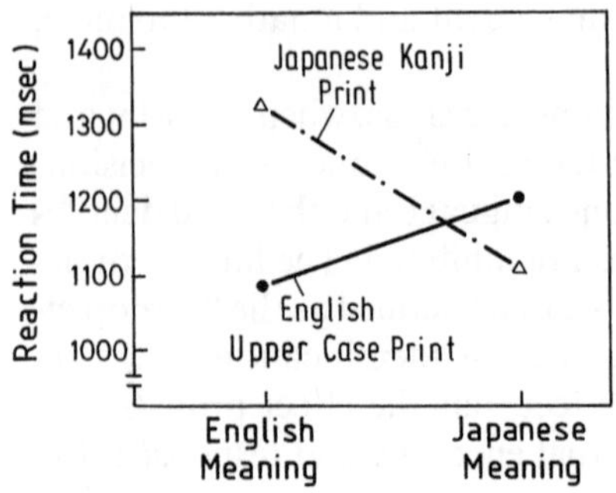

Fig. 4. The "Stroop effect" in the bilingual experiment, showing faster responses when the print and meaning match and slower responses when the print and meaning are in conflict. The Stroop effect can be defined as mean difference RT (or accuracy) between the conflicting (incongruous) and matching (congruous) conditions

Finally, a differential "net effect" occurred in the two hemifields as a function of print type. In the RVF (Fig. 5) meaning decisions are in general faster than print decisions, but as the English type becomes more esoteric, print decisions become relatively easier and meaning decisions relatively more difficult. Moreover, the advantage of meaning over print decisions is greater for Kana than for Kanji, consistent with LH specialization for lexical semantic access in Kana. In the LVF (Fig. 6) there is a tendency for print decisions to be faster than meaning decisions, especially relative to the LH. As the English type becomes fancier, again print decisions become easier relative to meaning decisions, and more so than in the LH. Finally, Kanji shows an advantage of meaning over print decisions (which is larger than in the LH), whereas Kana shows and advantage of print over meaning decisions, contrary to the LH. This pattern is consistent with RH specialization for lexical-semantic access in Kanji.

The interaction of the net Stroop effect in the different scripts with the visual field of presentation provides processing dissociation confirmation of direct access in this task.

Thus, both hemispheres yield Stroop effects, though to differing degrees, reflecting the relative speed of print and meaning decisions for each type in each hemisphere. In this case automatic facilitation and inhibition occur in each side, suggesting a similar processing sequence whose bilateral components differ in relative efficiency.

The bidirectional interference observed here contrasts with the unidirectional interference observed in the classical Stroop color–word experiment. There, access of the meaning of the color name interferes with naming the color of the stimulus much more than vice versa. Unlike the standard Stroop experiment, ours involves nonverbal responses, and the mutual interference most probably reflects parallel processing of perceptual and conceptual information as well as competition for response selection. Here, a faster, more dominant process will put earlier and greater demands on available resources, thus creating greater interference with a slower, less dominant process than vice versa.

The data reported here on RH specialization for processing Kanji script and LH specialization for processing Kana script need not mean that normal

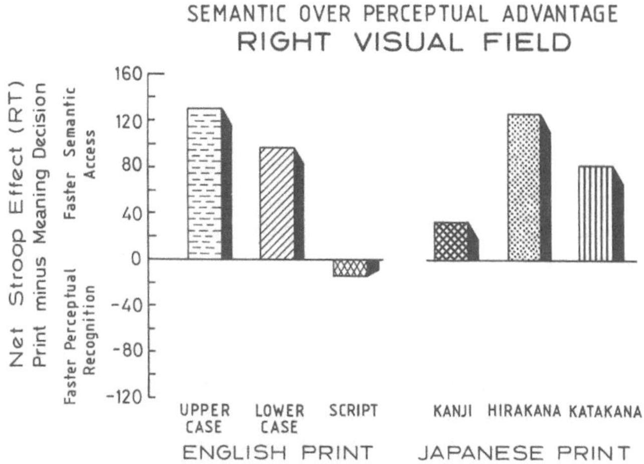

Fig. 5. "Net Stroop effect" for the various print types in the right visual half-field, showing the difference between the Stroop effect for print decisions minus the Stroop effect for meaning decisions (see Fig. 4). The net Stroop effect can be regarded as a measure of speed of lexical access relative to perceptual identification

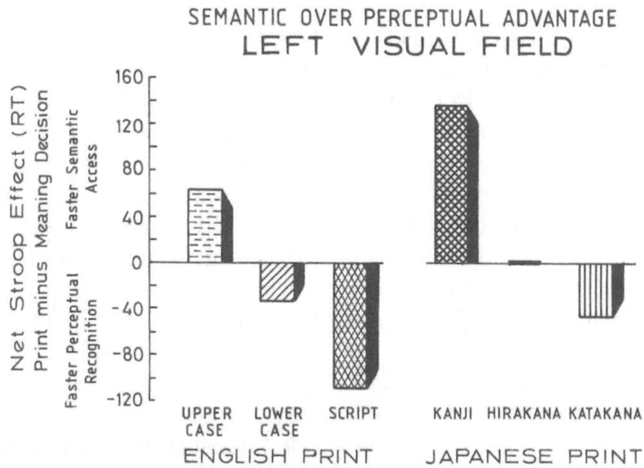

Fig. 6. Net Stroop effect for the various print types in the left visual half-field. See Figs. 4 and 5 for an explanation

reading of these two scripts is necessarily controlled by different hemispheres. But the data do show that perceptual analysis and semantic access occur automatically and independently in each hemisphere, and that the RH is better in perceptual than semantic analysis, whereas the LH is better in semantic than perceptual analysis. This means that the RH is not just competent to analyze printed words but that it is also ready to do so, in the sense that the requisite operations occur in it spontaneously and quickly. Active interhemispheric inhibition is required to stop lexical processing in the RH from proceeding to completion and controlling response.

Lateralized Semantic Priming of Lexical Decision

A study dealing with lexical decision and semantic facilitation was carried out by E. Zaidel, A. Radant and C. Temple (Zaidel et al. 1988). The lexical decision lists were developed by Allen Radant for his senior honors thesis at UCLA and included 128 pairs of prime and target letter strings. The primes and half of the targets were all highly imageable, concrete, and frequent words. The other half of the targets were orthographically regular nonwords. Half of the word targets were highly associated with their primes and half were not. An equal number of associated target word pairs (eight), unassociated target word pairs (eight), and target nonword pairs (sixteen) was assigned to each of four presentation conditions: (1) prime in the LVF and target in the LVF (LL); (2) prime in the RVF and target in the LVF (RL); (3) prime in the left and target in the right (LR); and (4) prime in the right and target in the right (RR). A go/no–go paradigm was used requiring speeded right-hand presses to word targets.

Two tasks were used: (1) targets alone. In this task no primes appeared. Subjects had to decide whether 50 ms targets spelled English words; and (2) visual priming. In this task a prime was flashed for 100 ms to one visual field and following an interstimulus interval of 500 ms, the target was flashed for 50 ms. Subjects were instructed to fixate a central fixation dot, ignore the prime, and respond to the target as fast and accurately as possible.

In each of the four conditions (LL, LR, RL, RR) the difference between the "targets only" and "primes plus targets" tasks may represent inhibition of the target by the unassociated prime and facilitation of the target by the associated prime. Figure 7 plots the difference in RT between the targets only

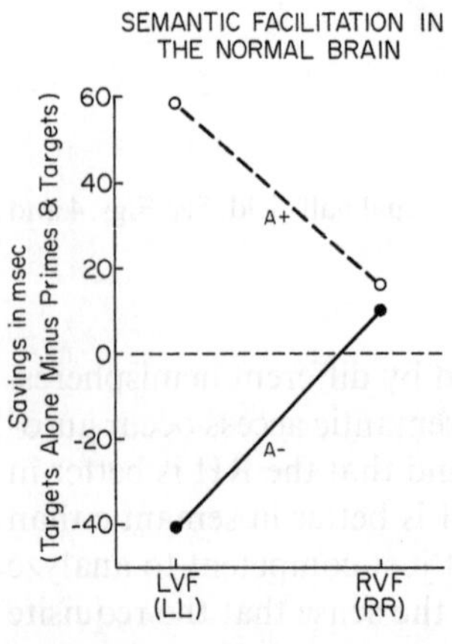

Fig. 7. Facilitation by associated primes and inhibition by unassociated primes in a lateralized lexical decision task administered to normal subjects. The *ordinate* describes the latency difference between lexical decision with the targets alone (no primes) and lexical decision with the same targets preceded by either associated (A+) or unassociated (A−) primes. A positive score indicates facilitation and a negative score indicates inhibition. *LVF* refers to the condition where both primes and targets are flashed in the left half-field (*LL*), whereas *RVF* refers to the condition where both primes and targets are flashed in the right half-field (*RR*)

and primes plus targets in the unassociated (A−) and associated (A+) conditions as a function of processing hemisphere (LL = RH, RR = LH). The figure illustrates a classic processing dissociation, indicating direct access. It shows that there is no inhibition and little facilitation in the normal LH, but strong inhibition and even greater facilitation in the normal RH. Thus, for this test at least, the primary locus of both the priming and interference effects is the normal RH! Automatic spreading activation for word association along the lexical-semantic network seems stronger in the RH than in the language-specialized LH, and this result is consistent with the view that there is a separate and differently organized lexical network in each hemisphere. The role of the RH network in normal natural language processing remains to be documented.

A Lateralized Comparative Judgment Task

In two experiments subjects saw (Experiment 3) a central comparative adjective (BIGGER or SMALLER) or heard it read aloud (Experiment 1) followed by two lateralized animal names (e.g., SHEEP and DEER) taken from a size-graded series (e.g., ant, ..., whale). Subjects were required to push a button corresponding to that member of the lateralized pair of animal names that matched the central or heard adjective. Thus, the sequence BIGGER followed by HIPPO, WHALE would require the subject to press the button corresponding to WHALE. In half the trials the comparative adjective and animal sizes represented the same pole of the dimension, e.g., BIGGER – HIPPO, WHALE (congruent pairs) and in half the trials the comparative adjective represented the opposite pole of the animal size, e.g., BIGGER – MOUSE, RAT (incongruent pairs). In Experiment 2 digits from 1 to 9 were used. These experiments were conducted by Dr. Hedy White while a postdoctoral scholar at UCLA and are fully reported in an article under submission (White et al. 1987). Pairs were lateralized pseudorandomly to the left and right visual hemifields, and the response hand was varied within subjects in counterbalanced blocks.

It is well established that congruent pairs are processed faster and more accurately than incongruent ones. Does this congruity effect occur in each hemisphere? In all three experiments there were significant response hand × visual hemifield interactions (with an ipsilateral advantage, i.e., best performance in the RVF-R hand and LVF-L hand conditions) for congruent pairs. This suggests direct access processing of congruant trials (see pp. 72,,73). However, incongruent pairs showed variable hand × field patterns suggesting direct access (contralateral advantage, i.e., best performance in RVF-L hand and LVF-R hand conditions due to interference between central processing and response programming) in one experiment, a callosal relay with LH specialisation in another, and a callosal relay with RH spezialization in the third. Thus, in the two latter experiments, where congruent pairs are processed in either hemisphere but incongruent pairs require specialized or unilateral hemispheric processes, the apparent comgruity effect reflects interhemispheric interaction and is partly due to callosal transfer.

Experiment 1, Animal Names. In this experiment the comparative adjective was read aloud and the animal names were drawn from four graded four-term series and included intermediate (i.e., neither congruent nor incongruent) pairs. Sixteen right-handed male and sixteen female UCLA undergraduate students participated in this experiment. Figure 8 shows the hand × field RT interactions for congruent and incongruent pairs of animal names in the first experiment for male subjects only. Congruent pairs show a direct access pattern but incongruent pairs show a callosal relay pattern with RH specialization. Thus only the RH seems able to process both types of pairs and only it could therefore be a unilateral source of the congruity effect. That is, if the "locus" of the congruity effect were to be in a single hemisphere and the effect were not to involve interhemispheric interaction or callosal transfer, then the only candidate for it in this experiment would be the right hemisphere. For, only the right hemisphere could process both congruent and incongruent pairs and only it could therefore (even in principle) then show a latency difference constituting the congruity effect.

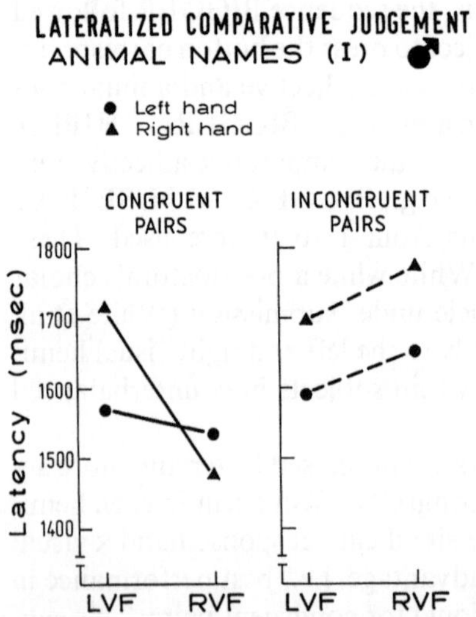

Fig. 8. Experiment 1. Pattern of latencies of the normal male subjects only for all pairings of visual half-field of presentation and response hands in a visually lateralized comparative judgment task with unimanual responses and animal name stimuli. Subjects signal manually the member of a pair of lateralized animal names (e.g., HIPPO, WHALE) that corresponds to a centrally presented adjective (e.g., BIGGER). *Congruent pairs* refer to trials in which the pair of animal names is from the end of the series (e.g., SMALL) that corresponds to the adjective (e.g., SMALLER – MOUSE, RAT?). *Incongruent pairs* refer to trials in which the pair of animal names is from the end of the series (e.g., BIG) opposite to the adjective (e.g., SMALLER – HIPPO, WHALE?). The visual field × hand pattern suggests direct access for congruent pairs but callosal relay, with right hemisphere specialization, for incongruent pairs

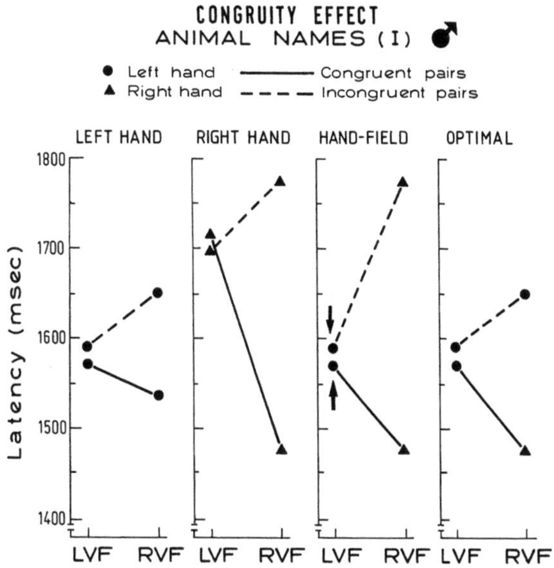

Fig. 9. Experiment 1. Latencies of responses to congruent and incongruent pairs of animal names by the male subjects only as a function of different possible combinations of visual half-field of presentation and response hand. Each *panel* represents an alternative potential interpretation of the congruity effect in each hemisphere (see text). The *arrows* indicate the most likely source of the real congruity effect if, as the data suggest, only the right hemisphere can process both congruent and incongruent pairs (see Fig. 8)

In Fig. 9 we plot the congruity effect in the two visual fields for various possible response hand combinations in this experiment. The "left-hand" panel may be interpreted to reflect the apparent congruity effects in the two visual half-fields if the right hemisphere controlled all decisions/responses. In that case, there would be no congruity effect in the LVF and, since it is assumed that the right hemisphere controls all decisions, the congruity effect in the RVF would be artifactual. The "right-hand" panel could be interpreted to reflect the apparent congruity effects in the two visual half-fields if the left hemisphere controlled all decisions/responses. This interpretation is clearly wrong in this experiment (see Fig. 8 and above) and yet it is the finding most neuropsychologists are likely to obtain since they collect only right-hand responses. The "hand-field" panel presupposes hemispheric independence and interprets the left visual field–left hand combination as right-hemisphere responses and the right visual field–right hand combination as left-hemisphere responses. In the optimal combination we plot for each field and type of word pairs the hand combination that yields fastest responses. The optimal panel again presupposes hemispheric independence so that left-hemifield presentations reflect right-hemisphere processing and right-hemifield presentations reflect left-hemisphere processing. In addition, the optimal combinations minimize response programming interference or callosal transfer effects by pairing each visual field with that hand that responds fastest.

If the congruity effect were to have two separate loci, one in each hemisphere, and if there were no interference between central processing and response programming in either hemisphere, then the panel most likely to reflect the separate congruity effects is the hand–field combination which pairs the field and hand controlled by the same hemisphere. If the congruity effect were to have an independent locus in each hemisphere but there was also interference between perception, processing, and responding in either hemisphere, then the panel most likely to reflect the separate congruity effect is the optimal combination, which is the same as the hand–field combination except for excluding interference effects when they are present (contralateral advantage). Thus, only the hand-field (LVF-L hand, RVF-R hand) and optimal combinations can be reasonably interpreted to reflect independent hemispheric processing and yet both show no congruity effect in the RH, which alone could give rise to it! All other apparent congruity effects are not directly due to semantic or symbolic properties of the stimuli and reflect in part delays in processing due to callosal transfer. In particular, the RVF-R hand combination, which most likely approximates the standard administration of the task, shows the largest apparent yet nonsymbolic congruity effect.

Experiment 2, Digits. In this experiment only congruent or incongruent (i.e., no intermediate) pairs of digits from the series 1,...,9 were presented. The comparative adjective was shown centrally. The hand × field RT interactions for congruent and incongruent pairs in experiment 2 show a direct access pattern for congruent pairs but a callosal relay pattern suggesting LH specialization for incongruent pairs (Fig. 10). Here, then, only the LH seems capable of processing both types of pairs and only it could therefore give rise to a unilateral congruity effect. The possible congruity effects for the two visual fields are plotted in Fig. 11 and the hand-field and optimal combinations do suggest a moderate congruity effect in the LH.

Experiment 3, Animal Names. This experiment attempted to replicate Experiment 1 using male subjects only. Here the comparative adjective was flashed centrally rather than spoken. The animal names were selected from one nine-term graded series and included only end terms, i.e., no intermediate pairs. There was a direct access hand × field pattern (Fig. 12) for both congruent pairs (ipsilateral advantage) and incongruent pairs (contralateral advantage reflecting interference between central processing and response programming within a hemisphere). Thus each hemisphere can process all information independently, including both congruent and incongruent pairs, and each can yield a separate congruity effect. Then the LVF-L hand condition may be said to reflect right-hemisphere processing, the RVF-R hand condition may be said to reflect left-hemispheric processing, and inspection of the hand-field panel

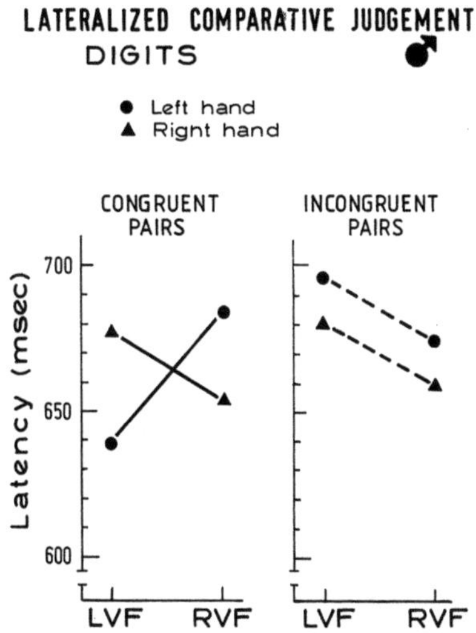

Fig. 10. Experiment 2. Latencies of responses by the male subjects only to a comparative judgment task with digit stimuli from the series 1, ..., 9, as a function of field of presentation and response hand. The data suggest a direct access pattern for congruent pairs (e.g., 7, 8 - BIGGER?) and a callosal relay pattern with left hemisphere specialization for incongruent pairs (e.g., 2, 3 - BIGGER)

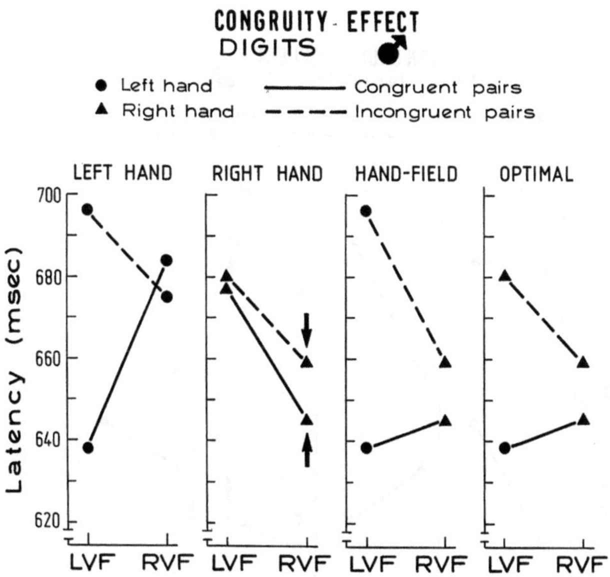

Fig. 11. Experiment 2. Latencies of responses by the male subjects only to congruent and incongruent digit pairs as a function of different possible combinations of visual half-field of presentation and response hand. The *arrows* indicate the most likely source of the real congruity effect since only the left hemisphere can process both congruent and incongruent pairs (see Fig. 10)

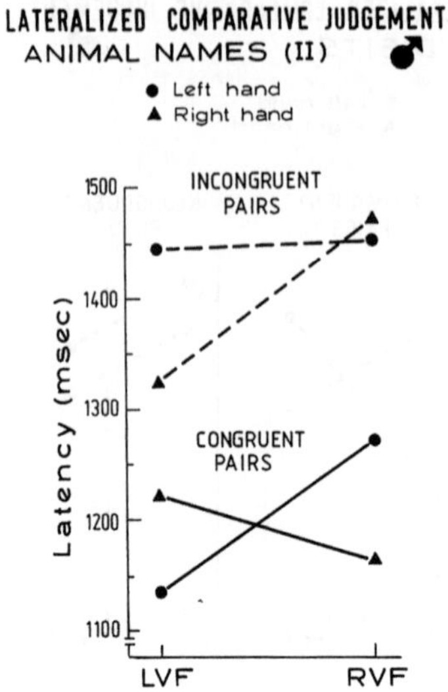

Fig. 12. Experiment 3. Latencies of responses by the all male subjects to a modified version of the comparative judgment task with animal names. Data shown for congruent and incongruent pairs as a function of visual half-field of presentation and response hand. The results suggest direct access for both congruent and incongruent pairs

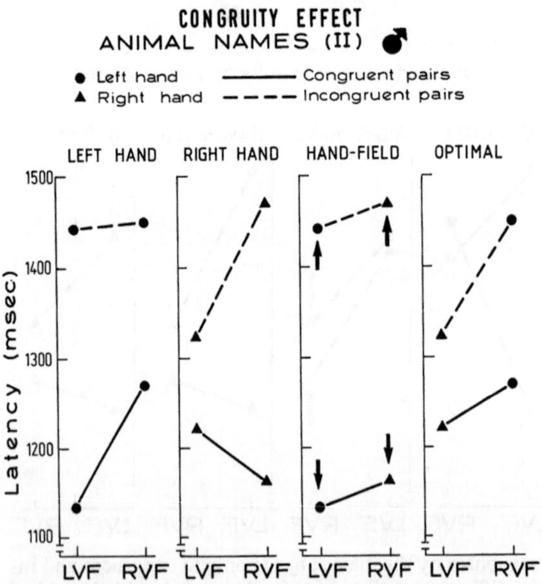

Fig. 13. Experiment 3. Latencies of responses by the all male subjects for congruent and incongruent pairs as a function of different possible combinations of visual fields and response hands. Since each hemisphere seems to process both congruent and incongruent pairs, the left visual field–left hand combination shows the congruity effect in the right hemisphere, and the right visual field–right hand combination shows the congruity effect in the left hemisphere. Both hemispheres then have similar congruity effects (*arrows*)

of Fig. 13 suggests that there is a large congruity effect in each hemisphere. Part of this effect is clearly not semantic or symbolic, however, since the latencies for incongruent pairs which show a contralateral advantage (i.e., faster responding with the RVF-L hand and LVF-R hand conditions), reflect in part some interference between processing and responding. (Recall that the congruity effect for a given condition is computed as the latency for incongruent pairs minus the latency for congruent pairs.) The optimal hand-field combination shown in Fig. 13 minimizes such interference effects and shows a larger congruity effect in the LH.

In summary, it is generally not the case that the two hemispheres show separate and independent symbolic congruity effects. In experiment 1 the LH could not have given rise alone to a congruity effect; likewise the RH in experiment 2. Furthermore, small changes in stimulus and task variables radically change the pattern of hemispheric involvement and the resulting congruity effect. Standard administrations of comparative judgment tasks are likely to further complicate the degree of each hemisphere's involvement with the task and consequently yield congruity effects that are at least partly attributable to hemispheric differences in processing congruent and incongruent combinations.

Discussion

Right-Hemisphere Participation in Language

Competence Versus Performance. Lateralized tachistoscopic experiments of the kind described in this paper can at best tap the limits of the lexical semantic competence of the normal right hemisphere. The data do not speak directly to the issue of right-hemisphere performance and participation in natural language processing. Systematic comparisons between hemisphere-damaged patients, patients with complete cerebral commissurotomy, and normal subjects surprisingly suggest that, of the three, the normal right hemisphere shows evidence for highest language competence. Normal subjects often demonstrate right-hemisphere involvement in tasks on which the disconnected right hemisphere fails (e.g., Zaidel 1983a; Eviatar et al. 1988). Aphasic patients, in contrast, often illustrate minimal right-hemisphere involvement, showing failure in the same lexical-semantic tasks competently performed by the disconnected right hemisphere (Zaidel 1986).

The one possible exception to the latter observation is the case of right-hemisphere speech in aphasia. Aphasics often do, and commissurotomy patients do not, show evidence for right-hemisphere speech. Perhaps speech is unique among language functions in requiring unified motor control, so that right-hemisphere speech competence is inhibited even in the disconnected brain through noncallosal influences though not in the aphasic brain with impaired speech centers.

In general, the possibility of dysfunction due to inhibition is present in any of the three populations and complicates the mapping of right-hemisphere language competence. However, although the reasons for this are still unknown, converging data suggest that such right-hemisphere dysfunction due to inhibition is minimal for lexical semantics. Indeed, data from commissurotomy patients and from aphasics as well as from normal subjects all suggest right-hemisphere ability to make lexical decisions.

Two Lexicons. Do the two hemispheres share the same lexicon with different access routes to it, or do they contain two separate and differently organized lexicons? The ubiquity of laterality differences in lexical semantics, involving numerous variables ranging from part of speech (Zaidel 1983 b), concreteness, and semantic field (Zaidel 1976) to emotionality and length (Eviatar and Zaidel 1988), suggests the existence of separate left- and right-hemisphere lexicons. Otherwise we would be forced to posit highly complex and specialized hemispheric access routes that embody much of the structure usually associated with the lexicon itself. Moreover, demonstrated hemispheric differences in lexical organization, such as graphemic-phonemic relations, are easier to account for in terms of structural differences in the lexicons than in terms of operations on a single lexicon. But, of course, these plausibility arguments remain only suggestive and speculative until a definite, complete, and coherent model of the lexicon is articulated.

What Is Right-Hemisphere Language for? A Proposed Role for Dynamic Hemispheric Interaction. We think of the two hemispheres as separate cognitive systems that process information in parallel and often independently. Each evaluates the environment and computes actions to solve particular problems. Overall interhemispheric control then assigns priority and effects integration. Thus, the right-hemisphere lexicon may help that hemisphere to integrate linguistic input into its model of the environment, affecting its evaluation of nonlinguistic actions.

Right-hemisphere contributions to natural language processing may in turn involve orientation to the context of communication. For example, it may help specify the semantic context in reading by processing connotative lexical meaning, on the one hand, and by integrating material across paragraphs, on the other. Most importantly, the right hemisphere provides a dynamic resource whose contribution to natural language processing changes continuously to optimize left-hemisphere analysis. In this view, the right hemisphere usually supplements left-hemisphere processing; sometimes right-hemisphere processes are recruited to replace otherwise engaged left-hemisphere mechanisms; other times the right hemisphere monitors what the left hemisphere had processed (Zaidel 1987).

Neuropsychologic Reinterpretation. It is possible to order lexical psycholinguistic effects along a complexity scale from those due to basic and mandatory processes shared by both hemispheres, through those that reflect more sophisticated processes specialized in one hemisphere, to those most advanced that require interhemispheric interaction.

The Stroop-like interference between automatic visual and lexical-semantic analysis occurs in both hemispheres, but the relative timing of the two processes is different in the two hemispheres and different scripts yield different relative effects in the two sides. Performance of this task in central vision can then reflect takeover of control by one hemisphere, depending on the stimuli and varying across individuals.

Associative priming and inhibition of lexical decision of concrete nouns, on the other hand, reflects predominantly RH processing, and failure to show the effects in central vision may result from LH takeover in some individuals. Chiarello's results (this volume) show that this finding too may be limited to a narrow paradigm or stimulus set. Right-hemisphere dominance, yet again, seems to be labile and very sensitive to stimulus, task, and subject variables.

Finally, congruity effects in comparative judgment can be "epiphenomena" attributable to callosal transfer required for specialized hemispheric processing of incongruent pairs. Thus the effects are not exclusively semantic. Since these congruity effects often reflect complex interhemispheric interaction under conditions of unilateral presentations, they are also likely to reflect such interactions, with all the attendant nonsemantic contributions, in central presentations, which is the standard cognitive psychological paradigm for this task. On the other hand, these congruity effects appear to be inherently labile and change radically as a function of stimulus and task demands.

Acknowledgements. Thanks to Chris Chiarello and Bill Milberg for helpful comments on the manuscript.

References

Eviatar Z, Zaidel E (1988) Effects of length and emotionality on hemispheric decisions of abstract nouns. (submitted for publication)

Eviatar Z, Menn L, Zaidel E (1987) Right-hemisphere contribution to lexical analysis. (submitted for publication)

Sakurai E, Zaidel E (1988) Japanese-English stroop effects with print and semantic decisions demonstrate hemispheric independence for automatic processing in the normal brain. (in preparation)

Stirling N (1979) Stroop interference: an input and an output phenomenon. Q J Exp Psychol 31:121–132

White H, Banks WP, Zaidel E (1988) Laterality effects in symbolic judgment: the influence of semantic congruity on hemispheric processing. (submitted for publication)

Zaidel E (1976) Auditory vocabulary of the right hemisphere following brain bisection or hemidecortication. Cortex 12:191–211

Zaidel E (1983a) Disconnection syndrome as a model for laterality effects in the normal brain. In: Hellige J (ed) Cerebral hemisphere asymmetry. Praeger, New York, pp 95–151

Zaidel E (1983 b) On multiple representations of the lexicon in the brain – the case of the two hemispheres. In: Studdert-Kennedy M (ed) Psychobiology of language. MIT, Cambridge, MA, pp 105–125
Zaidel E (1988) Lexical decision and semantic facilitation in the split brain. (submitted for publication)
Zaidel E (1985) Language in the right hemisphere. In: Benson DF, Zaidel E (eds) The dual brain. Guilford, New York, pp 205–231
Zaidel E (1986) Callosal dynamics and right-hemisphere language. In: Lepore F, Ptito M, Jaspers H (eds) Two hemispheres – one brain. Liss, New York, pp 435–459
Zaidel E (1987) Hemispheric monitoring. In: Ottoson D (ed) Duality and unity of the brain. Macmillan, Hampshire, pp 247–281
Zaidel E, Radant A, Temple C (1988) Individual differences in lexical decision and semantic facilitation within and across the hemispheres. (in preparation)

Representation, Control and Interaction: What Would a Theory of Right-Hemisphere Lexical Semantics Look Like? *

William Milberg

The axiom that there is only one cortical structure (or area) for each higher cognitive function and one function for each structure (with little or no redundancy) underlies much of neuropsychology and behavioral neurology. This, however, is only the simplest of a number of scenarios of how neural structure and cognitive function could in principle be correlated. The cortex might have been organized so that every structure subserved every mental function (e.g., as argued most recently by Lashley 1929). Alternatively, some structures could have subserved many functions or many structures could have redundantly subserved a single function. Each of these possibilities present special problems for the explanation and description of the effects of brain damage on behavior. The problems, however, associated with these latter more complicated principles of localization have up until this point been largely avoided in the study of the function of language. This is because language has been assumed to be the exclusive purview of the left cerebral hemisphere.

There can be little argument that the left cerebral hemisphere in most right-handed adults is of critical importance in all aspects of linguistic competence. However, as the chapters in this book attest, the right hemisphere appears capable of playing a role in the processing of metaphor (Bronell this volume), automatic access to subtle word meanings (Chiarello this volume), late access to word meanings (Joanette and Goulet this volume) and various aspects of reading as discussed in this volume by Weniger et al., Landis et al., and Zaidel et al. It appears then, that the view that a single cerebral hemisphere is exclusively responsible for language cannot remain unchallenged. This view at best is likely to be simplistic and at worst is likely to be a distortion of how the brain mediates higher cognitive activities. With increasing force the data from both normal and clinical populations seem to mandate that models of neural language implementation take into account the participation of a diverse set of separate and possibly multifunctional structures. Although it is premature to attempt to integrate this information into a single neuropsychological model of language processing, it is possible to discuss the "next generation" of questions posed by an emerging body of increasingly complex data.

There are a number of reasons why it is advantageous to construct a theoretical account of the neural implementation of a function, such as language, that implicates only a single hemisphere (and a strict model of functional lo-

* This research was supported by VA Merit Review 097-44-3765-001 to William Milberg.

calization). The evidence for the right hemisphere's direct participation in the function of language must be weighed against these advantages. It is obvious that under the assumption that "language" is localized in a single site (dedicated to that function alone), one greatly simplifies the enterprise of constructing maps of cortical functions and specifying how physically separated neural structures interact. Moreover, not only are the rules for mapping function on structure greatly simplified, but the advantages of studying language as an isolated modular system are obtained. Fodor (1983) has argued that those systems that operate autonomously with a set of automatically applied rules defining input/output relations are most likely to have a clearly defined biological status and are most likely amenable to scientific analysis. Under the assumptions of modularity, information used by one process cannot usually be used directly by another (e.g., information about light intensity cannot by used directly by the auditory system). A modular information processing device or system is encapsulated so that only its end product or output is available to other processing systems. Modular systems function as black boxes whose internal workings are opaque to consciousness. The processes within a module can operate without interference by other systems. Language, which is characterized by highly regular (but often opaque) rule-bound relationships between syntax, phonology, and meaning, is often considered to be an example of a higher cognitive function that is modular. In assigning the right hemisphere a role in lexical semantics (or any other aspect of linguistic processing) one must confront the question of its relationship to the other language processing devices of the brain: Does the right hemisphere engage in lexical-semantic processing as an autonomous system or as part of a single language processing device? The answer to this question is central to the interpretation of the data in the current volume.

First, a few more comments about neural information processing systems in general. Recent models attempting to capture the characteristics of human cognition often distinguish between the form in which information or knowledge is stored (henceforth: representation) and those processes which are used to access or manipulate that information (henceforth: control). This distinction does not necessarily imply separate neural hardware corresponding to each function. Indeed, the neural structures used for the representation of information might also participate in the "control" of that information. For the purposes of the current discussion, representation and control should only be considered as logically separable functional categories into which all cognitive processes can be classified. This distinction can be used to describe the possible relationships between two apparently separate neural processing systems.

Figure 1 summarizes four possible ways in which two processing systems that appear to be functionally different could interact. For two processing systems to be considered modular in organization, by definition both control and representational processes must be separate or isolated from each other. Because only the output of each system is available for further processing, communication between these systems is only possible via a third function. This

CONTROL \ REPRESENTATION	SHARED	INDEPENDENT
SHARED	Single Integrated Cognitive System (non-modular)	Quasi-Modular Cognitive System?
INDEPENDENT	Quasi-Modular Cognitive System?	Separate Cognitive Systems (modularity preserved)

Fig. 1. Possible interaction of two processing systems

third function must have the capability of recognizing and integrating their respective end products. In contrast, two processing systems that share representations and control would be considered to be completely nonmodular (or part of a larger modular system encompassing both). Attention is sometimes given as an example of a nonmodular function because it can affect how the outcome of most other cognitive processes is used.

Intermediate cases that are ambiguous with respect to the criteria for modularity can also be imagined. The first of these cases is a system where a single control function uses different kinds of representations. For example, a single lexical retrieval system might be used for both abstract and concrete words. Though both forms of words may be stored in different semantic formats (e.g., Paivio 1969), both have lexical forms that can be used referentially by a common phonologically based response system. In this example the criterion of informational encapsulation or specificity may have been violated at the semantic level, but preserved at the lexical level.

It is also possible that different control mechanisms use the same set of representations. Hughlings Jackson (1874) described the famous example of words that are uttered as part of an emotional response or as part of a propositional linguistic response. The word "damn" can be used reflexively as part of a response to pain or as part of a highly abstract utterance ("Damn the torpedoes, full speed ahead"). Hence, patients with severe aphasic symptoms can sometimes use such stereotypical words or phrases when emotionally aroused.

The ability to utter "a mighty oath" is unfortunately only a trivial example of different control functions using apparently similar representations. The issue of shared versus separate control, however, is not a trivial one. What happens if there is a conflict between the processing outcomes of the two control mechanisms? Which one will predominate in the response of the overall system? If the winner of the conflict is selected randomly, how can the system be made to function predictably? If one control system always wins the conflict, why waste limited resources on a nonfunctional system? Having two independent control processes for a single set of representations is therefore inherently inefficient and even dangerous (see Kosslyn 1987 for a more detailed presentation of a similar argument). Perhaps with unlimited processing resources a complex scaffolding of additional executive processes could be erected to decide which processor will ultimately control a response. With inherent biological limitations on space and speed such a system seems extremely unlikely. The problem of neural limitations of speed becomes critical when processing systems that are working on a similar problem are separated interhemispherically, as would be the case if the right hemisphere contributed directly to language processing. Initial processing time and interhemispheric transfer time must be fast enough to sustain the actual speed at which a particular function is performed on-line. This is an issue that can be determined empirically, but in many cases the speed at which an actual language processing task is performed will turn out to be faster than the limits of cross callosal transfer speed will allow. Localized control of processing is probably a biological response to the need to control processing rapidly and efficiently. In fact one could surmise that those functions that call for the most rapid input/output translations are those that are most likely to be neurally localized and lateralized. Modular organization of cognitive functions may then be a response to these biological limitations.

The problem of separate control functions can be avoided if the two different functions *only appear* to be using similar representations (and therefore performing an identical task) because the "surface form" of two different representations are similar. These surface representations may be the end products of two very different processing systems. One can use a computer graphics program to draw a perfect twelve point pica letter A that would in turn be totally unrecognizable by a computer word processing program using a similar looking font (Pylyshyn 1986). The control processes needed to create and recognize each letter are quite different, and the underlying representations of each letter is also quite different even though they appear to be similar on the computer screen. The graphic letter A is simply part of a field of light and dark shading with no inherent status as a letter, while the word processor letter A will be treated as part of an equivalent class of symbols with specified relationships with other symbols (e.g., "A" and "a" will be treated equivalently by a word processor). In this computer analogy modularity (and localized control) is completely preserved even though the end products of both systems can be made to look identical. The preserved ability of the aphasic patient to curse or to sing may simply be an example of two completely different processing systems (i.e., different control mechanisms using different representations) employing the same output channel (i.e., vocalization).

Finally, it is possible for a biologically limited neural system to homologously duplicate its functions. Under some circumstances homologously duplicated processing systems might even be advantageous. It is a common strategy for engineers to build duplicate back-up systems when the cost of failure of the main system would be great (e.g., airlines often have three radar systems). Such redundant back-up systems would be available if the main system were destroyed or overcommitted. To avoid the problems of intermodular conflict the back-up system would have to be ignored or deactivated until needed.

Although quite costly in terms of neural resources, some highly important systems (e.g., language) might justify such a homologous back-up. Centralized control and modularity are both preserved because the back-up systems do not functionally duplicate the main processing system; they only have that potential. In some cases processing systems may be duplicated adventitiously. That is, some or all of the processes that are controlled or represented in one area may be duplicated in a second area but never used. In the course of evolution (or development) one processor can gain priority because of its proximity to other available processing resources, while the other processor is never accessed in the course of normal information processing. Consider the following analogy: even though better tasting chickens are available from France, a French restaurant in New York will usually choose to use chickens from New Jersey because they will be fresher, cheaper, and delivery is guaranteed. Though the chef learned to cook with chickens from France, the chickens from New Jersey are more practical in a New York restaurant. Hence, the second homologous processor may be left as a vestigial remnant of an earlier phylogenetic (or developmental) stage with little or no current functional status within the main processing system. It remains, but never gains access to the main encapsulated processing system which capitalizes on more readily available resources. Recall that the now vestigial pineal gland was part of the visual system, as was the appendix of the digestive tract.

Now let us evaluate some of the evidence of the right hemisphere's apparent ability to process lexical-semantic information. These abilities may either be taken as evidence that the right hemisphere participates in language processing (and therefore should be considered part of a language module) or in language-like processing as part of an entirely different information processing system. The right hemisphere may even be an autonomous lexical-semantic processing system with its own representational and control processes or may be part of a single processing system controlled elsewhere. A theory of right-hemisphere lexical semantics must begin by considering these issues.

A good indication that a consensus about the relationship between the right and left hemisphere's language responsibilities has not been reached is the seemingly contradictory use of similar explanatory constructs by different authors. For example, in discussing his Stroop experiments with Kana and Kanji, Zaidel concludes that "automatic facilitation and inhibition occur in each side (hemisphere)." In contrast, based on their word list generation experiments, Joanette and Goulet conclude that the main problem of patients with right-hemisphere lesions "lies in their less automatic or 'controlled' activation" of lexical information (implying that the right hemisphere participates in "controlled" language processing). Finally, based on the analysis of her lexical decision data Chiarello concludes that "automatic semantic activation takes place in either hemisphere, but that some aspects of controlled semantic processing depend on a normally functioning left hemisphere." In each case these conclusions are logically derived from carefully conducted and clever experiments and yet do not easily fit into a single model of language processing or hemispheric interaction. These interpretative discrepancies are in part due to differences in the subject populations studied (normals versus patients with cortical lesions) and experimental paradigms used. However, contradiction is almost guaranteed because the experiments are not initially derived from similar models of representation, control, and hemispheric interaction.

The theoretical commitments in terms of the current discussion underlying some observations in the present volume can be more easily placed than others. Let us review several examples. Joanette and Goulet suggest that the words generated after the initial moments in a semantically constrained verbal fluency task are the result of a controlled search through the lexicon. The relatively poor performance of the right-hemisphere patients during these latter moments is interpreted as a lowered efficiency of less automatic search processes. They therefore appear to conclude that the right and the left hemisphere share representations but are differentiated in the manner in which those representations are accessed or controlled. This interpretation is subject to the problems of separate control devices sharing representations discussed earlier. To preserve modularity one could hypothesize that the verbal fluency task does not implicate the usual processes involved in on-line searches of the lexicon when sentences are produced. Perhaps this is evidence of a back-up system or a lexical search function used for an entirely different purpose.

Brownell reports an imaginative set of experiments using judgement tasks to study right hemisphere patients' appreciation of metaphoric and denotative meaning. He concludes that the right hemisphere serves as a memory buffer sustaining alternative meanings not immediately used by the left hemisphere. At first glance this interpretation would suggest that the right hemisphere serves as an extension of the main language processing functions of the left hemisphere, perhaps sustaining a set of representations not available in the left hemisphere alone. If this is the case, the question is raised as to why the alternative connotative or metaphoric meanings are not also inhibited when the more literal meanings sustained by the left hemisphere are inhibited. It could be that the delay imposed by interhemispheric transfer time simply delays the inhibition, thus maintaining the left hemisphere as the sole control site for retrieving all lexical information no matter what the form or location of the available representations. Alternatively, the right hemisphere could have its own control operations used for retrieving its own representations. Brownell recognizes this latter possibility when he notes that the patients metaphor deficit could be due to some "post-comprehension processing abnormality." The latter interpretation places right-hemisphere lexical semantics into a system that is essentially separate from the main language processing system in the left hemisphere. This maintains modularity and appears to match better with the metalinguistic nature of the judgement tasks used.

Interestingly, the interpretative framework used by Brownell was similar to that of Chiarello, who employed a lexical decision/divided attention paradigm with normal subjects. The lexical decision paradigm requires much more rapid responding than the judgement tasks used by Brownell and is therefore likely to implicate different cognitive operations. Chiarello concludes that automatic activation of lexical information occurs bihemispherically with controlled semantic processing occurring exclusively in the left hemisphere and gives an eminently plausible account of how these processes could be used in normal language. Chiarello's interpretation fits quite directly into a model based on unilateral control in the left hemisphere with bilateral or shared representations. Unlike Brownell's procedures, which allow for the possibility of independent right- and left-hemispheric operations, the time frame of the lexical decision paradigm is much closer to the time frame in which words must actually be interpreted. If it can be demonstrated that the selection time for choosing primary and alternative meanings occurs within the time limits of lexical activation (currently unspecified) and interhemispheric transfer time (ranging from 5–50 ms depending on the type of information that is transferred, see Cohen 1982), this would represent a plausible example of the right hemisphere's participation in actual linguistic lexical-semantic operations. If the time to select alternative meanings is considerably less than these time limits (RH activation time + interhemispheric transfer time), then it is more likely that the activation of lexical information in the right hemisphere occurs as part of a different information processing system or as example of an adventitious process not integrated into any active cognitive operation.

A similar step is necessary to fully interpret some of the data presented by Zaidel. In one study he suggests that the right hemisphere is specialized for the lexical interpretation of the Japanese ideographic writing system Kanji, while the left hemisphere is specialized for the lexical interpretation of the Japanese phonotactic writing Kana. He bases this conclusion on small but consistent field advantages observed in a series of split-field studies with Japanese/English bilingual subjects. In the current framework it appears that Zaidel posits that Kana and Kanji are processed by completely independent systems, each with its own set of representations and control mechanisms. If this is the case, the question must be asked as to how the lexical interpretations based on Kanji interact with the grammatical and even phonological information (pronunciation) that must in many cases be simultaneously processed in the course of normal reading. Does Kanji have its own complete language system available to it, or does the interpretation of ideography occur within the context of the left hemisphere's language processing system? It is possible that Kanji is interpreted by the right hemisphere and then using a set of highly specialized interhemispheric transfer routines developed after much practice is integrated into the main flow of language information within the left hemisphere. However, it is also possible that the specialization of the right hemisphere, no matter how expert, is not used in normal reading. Instead, it may be that Kanji is processed by the left hemisphere in the course of normal reading operations. The data, after all, do not show a complete absence of processing of Kanji in the right field, just a left-field advantage. In the course of developing localized neural control of reading, some of the right hemisphere's expertise with ideography may be sacrificed for the ability to integrate Kanji reading with other linguistic operations. Again the split-field superiority for Kanji may only be evidence of an adventitious specialization.

Obviously we cannot currently choose the correct interpretation of this data. Hemispheric specialization is only one possible interpretation of the evidence indicating half-field superiority. The next step will be to test the evidence of hemispheric specialization against the theoretical limits suggested by the normal function in its normal context. This should be accompanied by an evaluation of the neural costs and benefits of positing independent versus shared underlying processes.

Using the framwork of resource theory to discuss their data, Weniger and her colleagues raise the possibility that both hemispheres have similar capabilities that are tapped differentially depending on the complexity of task demands. In terms of the current discussion this implies two different systems using similar representations and control processes. The questions raised by this scenario should by now be familiar: which system controls output or response production?; how are the results of conflicts between independent computations of each system reconciled?; and if both systems are used simultaneously, how can independent results be used within the real-time framework of the function in question?

Landis and Regard's model of interhemispheric inhibition and complementary specialization of the two hemispheres in different aspects of both orthographic decoding and lexical interpretation appears to clearly preserve the two hemispheres as independent modular systems. An alexic patient was shown to be able to derive meaning from words when he was prevented from reading with a letter-by-letter strategy. When he was allowed to employ his typical letter-by-letter strategy, he was unable perform even rudimentary lexical interpretations. They also present evidence to show that the right hemisphere has its own special emotional lexicon. Although it is not clear whether or not this right-hemispheric reading system is normally active, Landis and Regard contend that without special alterations in the usual balance of power between the hemispheres it does not directly influence left-hemisphere lexical access. By defining a set of control processes and representations unique to the right hemisphere they preserve the left hemisphere as the main locus of most normal reading processes.

What is the function of a system that uses iconic reading and is particularly sensitive to words with high emotional content? As I have outlined earlier, there are a number of general forms that the answer to this question might take, some of which make the right hemisphere an actual functional system and others which do not (see Zaidel's discussion of the right hemisphere's lexicon as a self-contained slave system in this volume for a fascinating possibility). Perhaps the evidence of the right hemisphere's sensitivity to emotional words (and even to metaphor as noted by Brownell, this volume) implies that lexical information interpreted by the right hemisphere affects language output indirectly at a more global level (i.e., over longer time periods) than lexical information interpreted by the left hemisphere (whose interpretations are immediate and direct). The ultimate destination of the lexical output of the left hemisphere may be a sentence, while the ultimate output of the right hemisphere may be a mood. This could be the mechanism underlying the emotional impact of poetry and song. In any case, by maintaining the right hemisphere as a modular processing system with its own set of representations and control processes, interesting possibilities are opened for interpreting its lexical-semantic competence.

This final observation suggests that a broad conclusion may be derived from our analysis of the innovative research reported in this volume: as a cautious starting point the right and left hemispheres should be assumed to be independent nonreduplicative processing systems. It is not enough to identify analogous capabilities in both hemispheres. The details of control, representation, and interaction must also be identified and tested against the limits imposed by the actual on-line performance of the function in question. In many, if not most, cases explanations retaining a complete separation of representation and control will be more plausible than explanations melding the hemispheres into a single system. However, cases will remain where functional interhemispheric interaction of control and representation is the best explanation.

These theoretical issues are complex, but should not be entirely daunting. The building blocks for developing a broad understanding of cortical functioning are provided by precisely documenting the incredible range of functions in which the right hemisphere can potentially participate. It is hoped that the reader is convinced that with some imagination the blueprint for constructing a theoretical framework to interpret this exciting body of new data will also become available.

Acknowledgements. Thanks to Patrick Kilduff, Nancy Hebben, and Gina McGlinchey-Berroth for their comments on earlier drafts of this manuscript.

References

Cohen G (1982) Theoretical interpretations of lateral asymmetries. In: Beaumont JG (ed) Divided visual field studies of cerebral organization. Academic, London

Fodor J (1983) The modularity of mind. MIT, Cambridge, MA

Jackson JH (1874) On the nature of the duality of the brain. Med Press Circ 19(1):41–63

Kosslyn SM (1987) Seeing and imagining in the cerebral hemispheres: a computational approach. Psychol Rev 94(2):148–175

Lashley KS (1929) Brain mechanisms and intelligence. University of Chicago Press, Chicago
Paivio A (1969) Mental imagery in associative learning and memory. Psychol Rev 76:241–263
Pylyshyn ZW (1986) Cognitive science and the study of cognition and language. In: Schwab EC, Nusbaum HC (eds) Pattern recognition by humans and machines, vol 1: speech perception. Academic, Orlando

Subject Index

[illegible]

[illegible] Publisher [illegible]

[illegible]

Springer [illegible] Customer Service [illegible]

[illegible] 3, 69115 Heidelberg, Germany

Printed by [illegible] GmbH,

in Hamburg, Germany

MIX
Papier aus verantwortungsvollen Quellen
Paper from responsible sources
FSC® C105338

If you have any concerns about our products,
you can contact us on
ProductSafety@springernature.com

In case Publisher is established outside the EU,
the EU authorized representative is:
Springer Nature Customer Service Center GmbH
Europaplatz 3, 69115 Heidelberg, Germany

Printed by Libri Plureos GmbH
in Hamburg, Germany